T0134080

"Sean's books are the industry standard for passing NABCEP exams. I teach NABCEP Associate classes and want my students to pass. Sean's book – *Solar Photovoltaic Basics* – is the primary text and study guide I utilize to assure my students' success."

– Spencer Wright, Solar PV Technical Trainer, Solar PV Inspector

Praise for the previous edition

"I took Sean White's Entry Level PV Course and passed the NABCEP Exam right away. He has a great way of explaining things. I recommend his book!"

– David Inda, Fleet Manager, Clean Power Finance

Solar Photovoltaic Basics

This book explains the science of photovoltaics (PV) in a way that most people can understand, using the curriculum which reflects the core modules of the NABCEP Associate Exam. Whether or not you are taking the NABCEP Associate Exam, learning the material covered in this book is the best investment you can make insuring your place and moving up in the solar industry.

Providing complete coverage of the NABCEP syllabus in easily accessible chapters, this book addresses all of the core objectives required to pass the exam, including the ten main skill sets:

- PV Markets and Applications
- Safety Basics
- Electricity Basics
- Solar Energy Fundamentals
- PV Module Fundamentals
- System Components
- PV System Sizing Principles
- PV System Electrical Design
- PV System Mechanical Design
- Performance Analysis, Maintenance and Troubleshooting.

You will learn the importance of surveying a site and how to carry out a survey, how to use the tools that determine shading and annual production, and the necessity of safety on site. This guide also includes technical math and equations that are suitable and understandable to those without engineering degrees, but are necessary in understanding the principles of solar PV.

This new edition of Sean White's highly successful study guide has been updated throughout and reflects recent changes in the industry.

Sean White is a Solar PV professor, trainer and contractor, and was the IREC Trainer of the year in 2014. Sean has worked with NABCEP on various projects and travels the world teaching PV classes in person and online. He is based in the USA.

Solar Photovoltaic Basics: A Study Guide for the NABCEP Associate Exam

Second Edition

Sean White

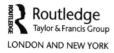

Routledge
Taylor & Francis Group
LONDON AND NEW YORK

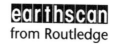

from Routledge

Second edition published 2019
by Routledge
2 Park Square, Milton Park, Abingdon, Oxon OX14 4RN

and by Routledge
711 Third Avenue, New York, NY 10017

Routledge is an imprint of the Taylor & Francis Group, an informa business

First edition published by Routledge 2015

British Library Cataloguing-in-Publication Data
A catalogue record for this book is available from the British Library

Library of Congress Cataloging-in-Publication Data
Names: White, Sean (Electrical engineer), author.
Title: Solar photovoltaic basics : a study guide for the NABCEP Associate Exam /
Sean White.
Description: Second edition. | Abingdon, Oxon ; New York, NY : Routledge, [2018]
Identifiers: LCCN 2018009746| ISBN 9781138102859 (hardback) |
ISBN 9781138102866 (pbk.) | ISBN 9781315103396 (ebook)
Subjects: LCSH: Photovoltaic power systems--Examinations--Study guides.
Classification: LCC TK1087 .W45 2018 | DDC 621.31/244076--dc23LC record
available at https://lccn.loc.gov/2018009746

ISBN: 978-1-138-10285-9 (hbk)
ISBN: 978-1-138-10286-6 (pbk)
ISBN: 978-1-315-10339-6 (ebk)

Typeset in Rotif
by Servis Filmsetting Ltd, Stockport, Cheshire
Printed and bound by CPI Group (UK) Ltd, Croydon, CR0 4YY on acid-free paper

Visit the eResources: https://www.routledge.com/9781138102866

Contents

List of illustrations

FIGURES

TABLES

Preface

Photovoltaics (PV) is a method of making electricity from light with a semi-conductor, usually silicon. Silicon is the same material from which a computer chip is made.

The solar industry is growing at light speed and now is time to get involved, to take part in reducing pollution and to take advantage of a great career opportunity.

By passing the NABCEP Associate Exam, you will have demonstrated that you are solar PV smart and ready to work in the fastest growing industry in the world.

This book is intended to help students learn the material on the exam in a reasonable time, while not getting overloaded with too much information. We will save the advanced material for another book, so you do not get overwhelmed.

Some of the more difficult material, such as voltage temperature calculations, will be covered multiple times in different ways throughout the book. This book is intended to be read and retained. Reading this book will be the most efficient time spent by busy people preparing to pass the NABCEP Associate Exam.

The NABCEP PV Associate Exam covers material, which is organized into ten learning objectives:

1. PV Markets and Applications
2. Safety Basics
3. Electricity Basics
4. Solar Energy Fundamentals
5. PV Module Fundamentals
6. System Components

7. PV System Sizing Principles
8. PV System Electrical Design
9. PV System Mechanical Design
10. Performance Analysis, Maintenance and Troubleshooting.

The chapters in this book will match the ten learning objectives.

There will be a special section at the end of the book focusing on voltage and temperature calculations, practice exam questions and definitions. And another practice exam with questions and answers can be accessed at www.routledge.com/Solar-Photovoltaic-Basics-A-Study-Guide-for-the-NABCEP-Associate-Exam/White/p/book/9781138102866

Once you master Photovoltaic Basics, it is time to take the next step to differentiate yourself. The most difficult NABCEP exam is the PV Installation Professional Certification Exam and we have a book for that, which is *Solar PV Engineering and Installation* by Sean White. Besides preparing students for the PV Installation Professional Certification Exam, the *Solar PV Engineering and Installation* book is recommended for those studying for the newer PV Inspector Certification Exam and the NABCEP PV Specialist Exams.

If your career is going to take you in the lucrative PV sales direction or if you just like to boost your resume with certifications, NABCEP has the Solar PV Technical Sales Certification exam and we have a book for that too, which is *Solar PV Technical Sales* by Sean White.

All of the NABCEP PV exams cover all of the material in this book.

The NABCEP (North American Board of Certified Energy Practitioners) Associate Exam was formerly known as the NABCEP Entry Level Exam. This exam was traditionally taken in Northern America, however with a breath of fresh air, NABCEP has taken a new direction and is has allowed Castle Worldwide Testing Centers to offer the exam at many locations around the world! NABCEP has gone global and is the worldwide "gold-standard" for renewable energy certifications!

For our international readers, there is a list of some common conversions and interpretations at the end of the book (Appendix 1).

Chapter 1

PV markets and applications

KEY CONTRIBUTIONS TO THE DEVELOPMENT OF PV TECHNOLOGY

1839: Edmond Becquerel discovered the photovoltaic effect.
1905: Einstein described the photoelectric effect and how light (photons) can excite electrons.
1922: Einstein received Nobel Prize for describing photoelectric effect.
1954: Bell Labs developed the "Bell Solar Battery".

> The "Bell Solar Battery" is what is technically called a solar module today.
>
> Often people incorrectly call a solar module a solar panel.

1958: First solar powered satellite sent into space by US Navy. The Vanguard 1 is currently the oldest man-made object in space.
1999: World total installed PV capacity 1 GW
> **1 Gigawatt = 1000 MW (megawatts)**
> **1 MW = 1000 kW (kilowatts)**
> **1 kW = 1000 W (watts)**

2012: World total installed PV capacity 100 GW, 31 GW of which was installed in 2012
2017: World total installed PV capacity over 300 GW
> **1000GW = 1TW. By the time many of you read this book, there will be 1TW of PV installed in the world.**

Figure 1.1 1956 PV advertisement from Bell Labs

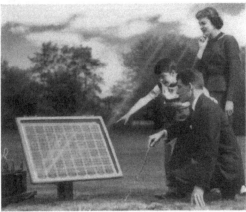

Something New Under the Sun. It's the Bell Solar Battery, made of thin discs of specially treated silicon, an ingredient of common sand. It converts the sun's rays directly into usable amounts of electricity. Simple and trouble-free. (The storage batteries beside the solar battery store up its electricity for night use.)

TYPES OF PV SYSTEMS AND THE BASICS OF HOW THEY OPERATE

GRID-TIED, AKA UTILITY-INTERACTIVE PV SYSTEMS

Grid-tied PV systems are connected directly to and synchronize with the utility. They are the most popular type of system. The **inverter is sized based upon the size of the PV array**.

The main components of a utility-interactive PV system are:

● Solar modules
● Inverter.

Self-consumption

We typically do not see batteries installed with interactive inverters, but times are changing and with an increased potential to overload the grid with solar energy in some places on a sunny day, there are reasons why batteries are added to an interactive system so that we will selectively have our inverters send out power, not just when it is sunny. When we have a system with batteries and the purpose is to operate when connected to the grid, we call this process self-consumption. Self-consumption systems are complicated and many solar installers try to avoid installing batteries. The purpose of self-consumption is to work when the grid is operating, as opposed to **battery-backup systems** which can operate when the grid is down. Some systems can do both self-consumption and battery backup. They say our car batteries will eventually be able to send out power to the grid. Exciting times!

Grid-tied PV systems have to be able to disconnect from the grid whenever the grid is down or not within specifications. This is called **anti-islanding** and means that the inverter cannot operate alone as an island of power. If a grid-tied system did feed the grid when the grid was down, it could be dangerous to utility workers who are fixing the problem. Some solar customers are surprised to find out that their utility-interactive PV systems will not work during a power outage.

Utility-interactive inverters are interactive inverters that work with the utility. Sometimes these interactive inverters are used in some micro-grid systems or other systems where there is no utility, so they are just called **interactive inverters** in the National Electric Code (NEC). A microgrid is a small grid of electricity and can be as small as your house or as large as a village.

STAND-ALONE, AKA OFF-GRID, SYSTEMS

Systems that work independent of the utility grid. Usually used for remote homes. Stand-alone systems are designed to fulfill all of the electricity requirements.

There are two basic types of stand-alone systems.

Direct current is the electricity from a solar module or a battery with a positive and a negative connection. Alternating current is what comes from your house and alternates very fast between positive and negative.

AC coupled systems   (ac = Alternating Current)
DC coupled systems   (dc = Direct Current)

DC coupled systems are the most common and simple off-grid systems. Their main components are:

● Solar modules
● Charge controller (prevents battery over- and under-charging)
● Battery
● Inverter.

AC coupled systems are complicated and less common. They use two types of inverters: **battery inverters** to create voltage so that **interactive inverters** can work when there is no utility. Their main components are:

● Solar modules
● Grid-tied inverters
● Off-grid inverter/charger
● Batteries.

Figure 1.2 DC coupled PV system

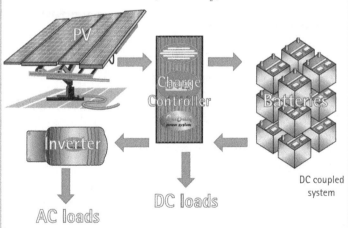

Stand Alone/Battery/Off-Grid

PV

Charge Controller

Batteries

Inverter

DC coupled system

AC loads

DC loads

The National Electric Code (NEC) aka "The Code"

The NEC includes the rules for installing safe PV systems. The NEC is published every three years, such as the years 2014, 2017, 2020, 2023 and 2026. Different places adopt different versions of the Code and often most of the solar installed in the USA is installed in places that adopt a version of the Code three years after it has been published. This book is not a book designed to teach you all about the NEC (we have other books for that). The NEC changed the definition of a PV system to not include batteries in the 2017 NEC. People always call solar modules solar panels and people will always call batteries part of the PV system; however we should mention this to give you an example of how the NEC evolves. If you are studying for the NABCEP Associate exam, have no fear, NABCEP is saving this complicated material for when you take the NABCEP PV Installation Professional Exam in the future.

HYBRID PV SYSTEMS

Hybrid systems include another source of power besides PV, batteries or the utility.

Typical other sources of power include:

- Generator (internal combustion engine)
- Wind turbine
- Micro-hydro (small hydroelectric turbine).

GRID-TIED-BATTERY-BACKUP

Multimodal systems can **operate as grid-tied systems and off-grid** systems. They are typically the most complex systems to design.

The inverters will typically produce as much power as possible when operating in utility-interactive mode. When the utility is interrupted, the inverters disconnect from the grid and switch to stand-alone mode and make as much power as the loads require. (**Loads are devices that consume electricity**.)

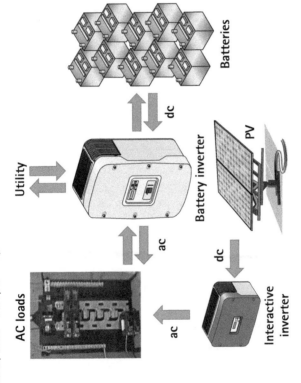

Figure 1.3 SMA Sunny Island AC coupled PV system

Multimodal systems have to disconnect from the grid completely when the grid is down, but still have to feed power to the building. These systems usually power a subpanel of specific loads and not the entire building.

Multimodal inverters

Multimodal inverters are inverters that can operate in multiple modes, such as interactive mode (connected to the utility) and stand-alone mode. These inverters are used for backup power for when the grid is down. Multimodal inverters are sometimes referred to as bimodal inverters.

DIRECT, AKA DIRECT-COUPLED PV SYSTEM

This is the **simplest type of PV system**. The **only components are PV and a load** (usually an electric motor).

A good example of a direct-coupled system is a solar attic fan. A solar attic fan consists of a PV module and a fan. When the sun is out, the fan works, when it is brighter, the fan works better, which is convenient, since we need a fan more when the sun is out.

Another common direct-coupled system is water pumping. In sunny times, more water is needed and water can be stored with elevation and used at night.

Direct water pumping system variation

Often times, water pumping systems use a linear current booster (LCB) which boosts current and sacrifices voltage at times of lowlight, such as mornings.

Informational note: You will learn later in this book that voltage x current = power and that power x time = energy.

There are no direct-coupled lighting systems, since when the sun is out the direct sunlight is the most efficient light. Perhaps modern-day cave dwellers could benefit from direct-coupled lighting systems.

SELF-REGULATING SYSTEM

A self-regulating system is a stand-alone system **without a charge controller**. In most cases, not having a charge controller would damage a battery by under- and over-charging the battery.

According to the National Electric Code, a self-regulating system has to be designed so that it will **not charge over 3% battery capacity in an hour**. This way the battery will not be over-charged. Over-charging a battery can not only damage the battery, but also can split water molecules into hydrogen and oxygen, which is an explosive combination (rocket fuel).

There are no safety issues with under-charging batteries, but as anyone with a car knows, letting a battery die is not good for the life of the battery, so self-regulating systems are designed with loads that are small relative to the size of the battery and PV, so that they can survive dark winter days.

A good example of a self-regulating system is a coastguard buoy, which has a big battery bank relative to a modest blinking light.

ADVANTAGES AND DISADVANTAGES OF PV

PV works when the sun is up and that is when people use electricity the most. We say that it generates at "peak" times, which makes it most valuable. Other conventional forms of energy production can be easily stored; however, when we are burning things to make electricity, we are doing something that causes pollution.

Wind power is good when mixed with solar, because wind can work at night, however most people would rather live in sunny places than windy places. Also, wind is intermittent, and sunshine is much more predictable. Even on cloudy days, solar systems make power. Solar works 365 days per year.

One of the problems that we have with solar is storage of energy so that we can use the solar energy at night. When solar was adopted early and solar energy was less than 1% of the energy produced on the grid, storage was not such a big deal; however, as the industry grows exponentially, storage becomes more important in places where solar is adopted to a greater degree. Energy storage is becoming more important in places where solar PV is more saturated, such as in Germany and Hawaii. As the need grows, production increases and the price drops with the development of new technologies. The price of PV has dropped tenfold in the last ten years. Battery prices are also dropping with mass production as are utility requirements for systems to refrain from exporting power to the grid at times.

When electricity is made where people live, we call that distributed generation (DG) and DG means that we do not have to transmit electricity over large distances. When electricity is transmitted, there are losses. Also, with electricity produced nearby, we do not have to pay for land and more infrastructure such as substations, high voltage power lines and transformers.

Utility scale solar farms are large solar projects, often in the desert where power is transmitted over long distances, such as is the case for most conventional power generation. This will add costs for substations and transformers, which often add millions of dollars to the project costs. Utility scale solar farms are often the fastest growing part of the industry due to economies of scale.

Most of the electricity in the world is made from coal. Heat from burning coal creates steam and that steam will spin equipment and make power. This is similar to the technology of a steam locomotive. Most people would rather live near a solar installation than a coal plant.

Nuclear power plants also use the heat of splitting radioactive material (fission) to make steam. As we know in the cases of Fukushima and Chernobyl, when we cannot keep the radioactive uranium cool, we can have a meltdown. Nuclear power plants can be difficult to turn off.

Burning natural gas is becoming popular due to the increased amounts of gas found using hydraulic fracturing (fracking). Fracking is controversial because of the effects on the water supply and because it is difficult to keep the small gas molecules from seeping out of the pipes. Some people think that natural gas is a good transitional fuel for solar while battery technologies are developing, since natural gas turbines can ramp up quickly as clouds come in front of solar arrays. Coal and nuclear take a while to ramp up.

Solar power is a safe form of nuclear energy. We are using fusion reactions that are 93 million miles away to make light (electromagnetic radiation) that we then convert to electricity with photovoltaic modules.

Much of the energy that we produce in the world is wasted and conserving energy is often a better value proposition than solar PV. One of the best energy investments one can make is an efficient light bulb. Better yet, natural sunlight makes light and a properly designed building can take advantage of sunlight for lighting, heating and cooling. Using architecture for solar energy is called "passive solar".

> PV on a rooftop can block sunlight from hitting the roof and keep a building cooler, lowering an air conditioning bill, even if the system is not turned on.

BENEFITS OF DIFFERENT TYPES OF PV SYSTEMS

Rooftop systems put the means of energy production on the roof, where energy is used, and protect the building from UV rays. Sometimes the building materials can be made from PV and this is called Building Integrated PV (BIPV). Since **BIPV is part of the building**, as is the case with a solar roof tile, then it will not have the same airflow underneath it as a regular PV system. When a PV system is hotter like this, the PV does not work quite as well as if it were operating cooler. **BIPV is not as efficient as regular PV because it is hotter** and it is more expensive, since regular solar modules are mass-produced to bring the cost down. BIPV also has more electrical connections for a given amount of power, which can be difficult to do maintenance on when the PV is part of the building. BIPV always gets a lot of attention and perhaps someday someone will figure out how to make BIPV financially feasible.

> Solar grid-parity is when energy produced by PV is less expensive than electricity produced by conventional means. Grid-parity is happening in different places in the world where there is a combination of factors, such as expensive conventional electricity, good sunlight (solar resource) and low installation and permitting costs. Hawaii and other tropical islands have expensive conventional energy and good sunlight. Germany has low installation and permitting costs. As more places reach grid-parity, mass production brings the price of PV systems down more and the grid-parity map grows!

Ground mounted PV systems are easy to install, but they take up valuable real estate and can have trouble getting permitted due to environmental restrictions.

Figure 1.4 97MW solar farm, Sarnia, Ontario, Canada
Source: Photo Sean White 2010. At the time, it was the world's largest PV system. System consists of approximately 1.3 million First Solar thin film PV modules.

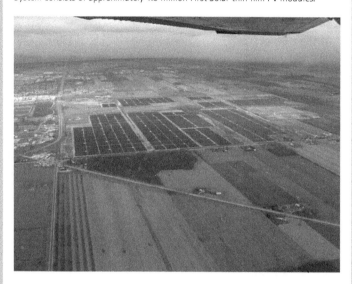

Safety basics

The two most common safety questions that you may run into on any construction-related exam have to do with fall protection. This is what you need to know:

1. **6 feet** is the height at which you need fall protection.
2. **1:4 ladder ratio.**

Figure 2.1 1:4 Ladder ratio

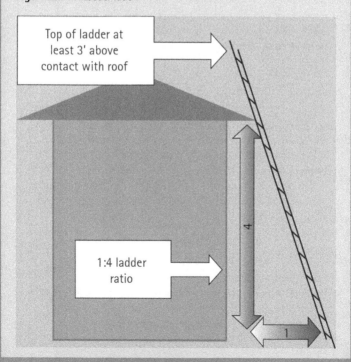

Top of ladder at
least 3' above
contact with roof

1:4 ladder
ratio

4

1

MORE SAFETY

Common sources for safety information are:

1. **OSHA** (Occupational Safety and Health Administration). There are federal and state OSHA requirements. State requirements cannot be more lax than federal.
2. **National Electric Code (NEC)**, which is published by the National Fire Protection Association (NFPA). The NEC is what electricians use to make sure their systems are safe. It is also what the **Authority Having Jurisdiction** (AHJ) will use as the rules to follow when inspecting electrical systems.

> The AHJ is typically the city or county building department or inspector for most PV projects, but also includes anyone who has jurisdiction over a project and can include the utility or the state. The AHJ will interpret the NEC and adopt a version of the NEC.

> The NEC will tell us which wire to use. If a lot of current flows through a wire, it will heat up. If it gets too hot, it will melt the insulation around the wire. If the wire is in a hot place, it can take less current than the same wire in colder conditions. The **ability of a wire to carry current is called ampacity**. The hard NABCEP PV Installation Professional Exam is an open book NEC exam. The exam will require test takers to use tables and difficult-to-understand code to demonstrate a working knowledge of wire sizing and PV design.

More ladder safety:

- Rungs (steps) of a ladder are about one foot apart.
- The ladder should be 3 steps (3 feet) above the top of the roof or object you are leaning ladder against.
- The ladder should be secured to the roof at the top.
- Painting a wooden ladder can be unsafe and hide ladder defects.

- Metal ladders conduct electricity so electrical workers should use heavier fiberglass ladders.
- Fiberglass ladders however have aluminum steps.
- Use an extension ladder to climb on a roof, not an A-frame ladder.
- Keep three points of contact on a ladder. Carrying objects up a ladder in one hand can be dangerous!

ARCING AND ARC FLASHES

Electrical **voltage is the hydraulic (water) analogy of pressure** and when voltage is higher, so is the chance of a spark or an arc.

In a PV system, if there is a small gap in a circuit, then we can have an arc where electrons will travel through the air. Many newer inverters are equipped with dc arc fault detection. If there is an arc, then the inverter should shut off. An arc is a "plasma discharge" and is a very hot fire hazard.

An arc flash is an explosion when a great amount of energy is released with an arc. When working with larger systems and close to the potential spark/arc, you need to have proper arc flash personal protective equipment, which is like a space suit. Arc flashes are hotter than the sun. Often the more dangerous source of power is the utility rather than the PV system. The utility has more potential than our PV systems.

> **PPE is personal protective equipment** and can include arc flash suits, earplugs, goggles, aprons and personal fall arrest systems (PFAS). PFAS are usually the most important types of PPE protection gear in the solar industry.

OVERCURRENT PROTECTION DEVICES

Fuses and circuit breakers are called overcurrent protection devices (OCPD) and are used to prevent fires. On the backside of a PV module, there is a label that says the **maximum series fuse rating**. The fuse will **open the circuit (turn off)** if there is too much current in order to protect wires and equipment. Not all circuits require fuses or circuit breakers.

Figure 2.2 Arc flash PPE
Source: Courtesy Honeywell

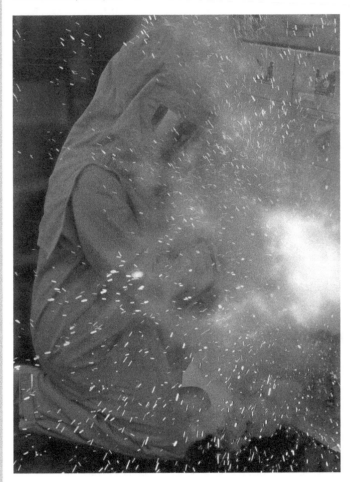

Figure 2.3 California Department of Public Health

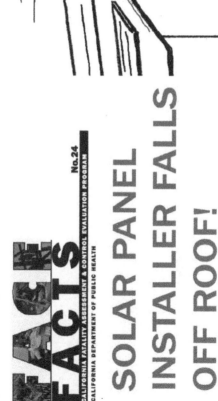

FALL PROTECTION

Falling is the number one cause of death in the construction industry.

Types of fall protection:

1. Guard rails
2. Safety nets
3. **Personal Fall Arrest System (PFAS)**.

The PFAS is the most common type of fall protection used in the residential solar industry.

PFAS consists of:

1. Harness
2. Shock absorbing lanyard
3. Lifeline
4. Anchor.

Figure 2.4 Harness
Source: Courtesy of Honeywell

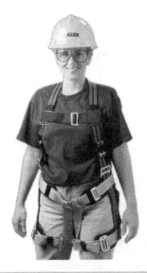

Figure 2.5 Shock absorbing lanyard
Source: Courtesy of Honeywell

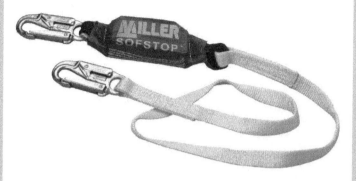

Figure 2.6 Anchor must hold at least 5000 lbs
Source: Courtesy of Honeywell

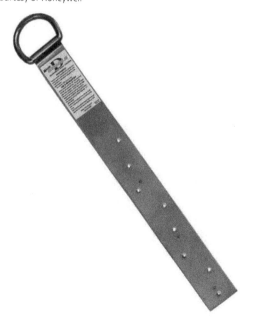

Figure 2.7 Keep the lifeline as short as possible
Source: Photo by Sean White at a very large solar factory near Shanghai China

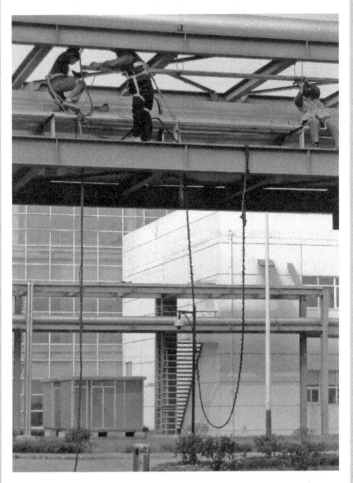

Figure 2.8 Fall protection must also be used around skylights. Skylights offer a false sense of security
Source: California Department of Public Health

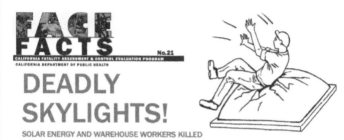

Figure 2.9 Two broken First Solar PV modules next to skylight where solar installer died
Source: California Department of Public Health

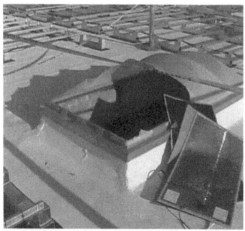

The skylight that the worker fell through

There are some types of PPE that are more important than other types. Fall protection is the most important PPE in the solar industry. Goggles are more important than an apron when working with lead acid batteries. Your eyes are more important than your clothes.

LOCKOUT–TAGOUT (LOTO)

When you turn off your solar system and then go on the roof, you want to make sure that you can lock the system in the off position, so that nobody turns the switch on and electrocutes you.

BODILY SAFETY

When you are working in the sun where there is no shade, protect yourself from the sun with sunscreen, drink plenty of water and wear a hat.

Also, with all safety precautions in place, people still get hurt and die, so above all, be extra careful!

Figure 2.10 Lockout-tagout kit
Source: Image provided Courtesy of Ideal Industries, Inc.

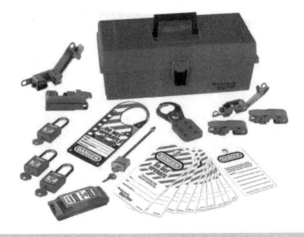

Electricity basics

In order to be competent with PV, we need to be competent with electricity.

Figure 3.1 Ohm's Law wheel

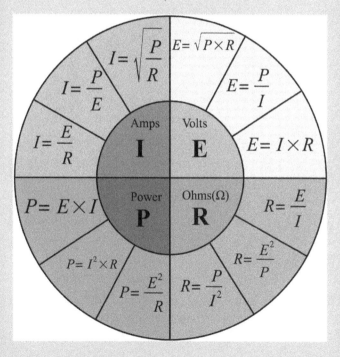

POWER AND ENERGY

Laypeople and even newspaper reporters often use power and energy interchangeably. This is not correct and is not the case for true solar professionals.

Power is a rate, just like speed is a rate.

Power × Time = Energy
Speed × Time = Distance

When we leave the lights on, the cost depends upon how long we leave the lights on.

Power is measured in watts and the way to remember that is that the middle letter in po**W**er is a W for Watts.

Just like 1000 meters is a kilometer, 1000 watts is a kilowatt or kW.

The metric system is used in the solar industry.

1,000 = kilo = k (thousand)
1,000,000 = mega = M (million)
1,000,000,000 = giga = G (billion)

We are just moving the decimal 3 places.

We talk about watts when we can speak of a 250W solar module.

When we talk about the twenty 250W modules on our rooftop, we will call that

20 × 250W = 5000W
5000W/1000 watts per kW = **5kW**

When we talk about bigger commercial PV systems, we can talk of 4000 250W modules

4000 modules × 250 watts per module = 1,000,000 watts
1,000,000 watts/1,000,000 watts per MW = **1MW of PV**

When converting, you are going to either multiply or divide by the conversion factor. It should be obvious if you multiplied instead of divided or vice versa. Make sure to use common sense rather than just memorization.

When we talk about the amount of solar in the United States, we will say that the US has over 13GW of PV operating as of 2013. That number usually doubles about every 18 months. In 2000 the world had about 1GW installed and in 2017, the world had over 300GW installed. With this growth rate, the world will be one giant solar array in 100 years!

> Be sure to fully understand the following definitions and relationships. Go back a few times a day if you have to. Bookmark this page or fold the corner.
>
> Repetition = memory.

Simple definitions:

- Voltage: Electrical pressure
- Current: Electrical flow
- Power: Rate at which electricity is used
- Energy: Amount of electricity used

Relationships:

- Power = Voltage × Current
- Energy = Power × Time

Units:

- Voltage is measured in Volts = V
- Current is measured in Amps = A
- Power is measured in Watts = W
- Energy is measured in Wh or more often kWh
    - pronounced <u>kilowatt hours</u> and not per hour!
    - a rookie mistake that makes you look inexperienced and would be very bad during a job interview is to refer to kWh as kW. Your electric bill at your house is for kWh not kW!

Symbols

- Current = I (I for Intensity)
- Voltage = V or E
- Power = P

Table 3.1 Electricity units and symbols

Phenomenon	Current	Voltage	Power	Resistance	Energy
Symbol	I	V or E	P	R	E
Units	Amperes	Volts	Watts	Ohms	Watt hours
Unit abbreviation	Amps or A	V	W	Ω	Wh

How to do the math required to be entry level PV proficient:

W = V × A

To solve for V, we put A under W

V = W/A

To solve for A, we put V under W

A = W/V

> Whatever symbol is alone in simple algebra will end up on top.
>
> If A × B = C then A = C/B and B = C/A
>
> C was by itself at first, so C is on top when solving for A or B.
>
> The next time you are lonely, just remember algebraically, loaners end up on top!

HOW TO CALCULATE ENERGY USAGE FOR AN OFF-GRID FOREST SERVICE FIRE LOOKOUT CABIN

You have a 12V 2A light bulb that will run for 3 hours per day.

You also have a 100W radio repeater that will be on 100% of the time.

How much energy in kWh does the cabin use in a day?

Answer:

12V × 2A = 24W

24W × 3 hours = 72Wh of energy per day for the lights.

100W × 24 hours per day = 2400Wh repeater

Total energy = 2400Wh + 72Wh = 2472Wh/day

Figure 3.2 Simple algebra triangle. This triangle works with all simple equations. Cover up what you need to solve for. In this example, I = P/V.
Source: Sean White

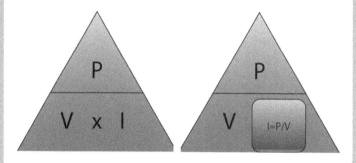

Convert to kWh

2472Wh/1000 Wh per kWh = 2.472 kWh

On a test or in real life, this could be rounded off to 2.5 kWh for the correct answer.

Remember that on the NABCEP tests, there are always four choices to choose from and you should make sure that your answer seems right. Remember that all good exam questions have wrong answers that were carefully thought out. Be careful of getting your units right and do not confuse Wh with kWh. You should have plenty of time to take the NABCEP Associate Exam, so do not rush. Make sure your answer makes sense. I like to take an educated guess at the range of right answers before I complete the problem. Another common mistake is moving the decimal in the wrong direction when converting kWh to Wh. Remember that when converting to large units, your final number will be smaller. Every time you do math, make sure your numbers make sense. Even the smartest people make simple mistakes. The smartest people will catch their mistakes. Try to not get lost in the math and make sure every step makes sense.

Common mistake:

Energy is kWh not kW/h or kW

BATTERY MATH

When talking about **battery capacity**, the term **Amp Hour** (Ah) is commonly used. An Ah is an amp for an hour. Amp hours are easily converted to Wh (energy).

Ah × V = Wh

A 6-volt battery that has 100 Ah has:

6V × 100Ah = 600Wh

A 12V battery with 100Ah has:

12V × 100Ah = 1200Wh

An easy way to convert Wh to kWh is to move the decimal 3 places.

kWh are bigger than Wh, so 1200Wh = 1.2 kWh

OHM'S LAW AND RESISTANCE

When power is consumed, we can talk about a relationship between current and voltage called resistance.

The relationship is called **Ohm's Law** and is:

V = I × R

This means that when current goes up and resistance remains constant, then voltage difference also increases. This is called a **proportional relationship**.

When current goes through a wire, there are losses and those losses are consumed by the wire in the form of heat. The losses are known as **voltage drop**. If the current is increased, so is the voltage drop/loss.

WHAT REALLY IS AN OHM?

An **ohm is a unit of resistance** also symbolized with the **Greek symbol** Ω.

Since $V = I \times R$ (We also can write $V = IR$)

Then $R = V/I$

> Since V was alone, it gets to be on top when I is put on the other side of the equation to solve for R.

We can say resistance is measured in volts per amp.

For entry level PV, we do not have to go very much deeper into resistance.

Let's do something fun with an inefficient 100W incandescent light bulb.

Practice question:

Using $W = VI$ and given that the voltage of the receptacle is 120Vac, how many Amps will be going through the light bulb?

Answer:

If $W = VI$ and we want to solve for I then

$I = W/V$
$I = 100W/120V$
$I = 0.833$ Amps

Therefore, next time you go to the store, ask for a 0.833A light bulb.

If they don't know what you are talking about, then try asking for your light bulb in Ohms.

Since V = IR then to solve for Resistance

R = V/I
R = 120V/0.833A
R = 144Ω

So ask for a 144 ohm light bulb.

Using W = VI and V = IR together, we can solve for W, V, I and R if we know any two of the factors. The Ohm's Law wheel at the beginning of this chapter gives derived equations to help electricians with this.

We could have looked at the Ohm's Law wheel and seen that:

$R = V^2/P$
$R = 120V^2/100W = 144$ ohms

HOW TO USE A METER TO MEASURE VOLTAGE, CURRENT AND MORE

Digital multimeters can typically measure voltage, current and resistance.

Figure 3.3 is an example of a simple and inexpensive meter that can measure voltage, current and resistance.

VOLTAGE MEASUREMENTS

Always turn the meter to a setting higher than you would ever expect to measure. The meter in Figure 3.3 has a red lead and a black lead that are used to measure voltage when the connectors are hooked up to the two out of three plugs on the right side of the meter. (When measuring current through the meter, the red lead will go to the left of the black lead.)

When measuring dc (direct current) voltage from PV or a battery, set the voltage to the setting with the solid line over the dashed line.

Figure 3.3 Digital multimeter

Source: Wikimedia Commons. Attribution: oomlout http://commons.wikimedia.org/
wiki/File:Digital_Multimeter.jpg. This file is licensed under the Creative Commons
Attribution-Share Alike 2.0 Generic license.

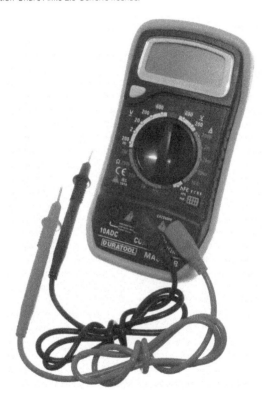

When measuring utility ac (alternating current), look for the symbol that looks
like this ~.

When measuring dc with the meter, the black lead of the meter is negative and
the red is positive. If you get red and black backwards, you will end up with a
negative number for voltage.

When measuring ac voltage, it does not matter if the red and black are one way or the other, since the voltage and current are constantly alternating on each side of zero.

MEASURING CURRENT

When measuring current with a multimeter as pictured in Figure 3.3, the meter will become part of the circuit and all of the current will run through the meter.

Most people in the solar industry would rather not have the current run through the meter for safety and simplicity.

We can also measure current without even touching a wire and this can be done with a clamp.

How to measure current with a clamp:

- Put the clamp around one wire in the circuit.
- Do not put the clamp around two wires in the circuit, such as in an extension chord. Every circuit is a circle with a return path and if you get two parts of a circuit, each with current going opposite directions, they will cancel each other out.

When measuring dc current with a clamp-on ammeter, make sure that you are either **clamping on the negative or the positive, but not both**.

Also, most clamp-on ammeters only measure ac current, so when you are shopping for clamp-on ammeters, make sure that you purchase one that has a clamp that works for dc, which is more expensive than an ac clamp.

MEASURING RESISTANCE AND CONTINUITY

Most digital multimeters can measure resistance and a good example of this is to measure continuity. Most meters will beep when there is a connection between negative and positive when they are set to measure continuity (continuity meaning continuous).

Figure 3.4 Digital multimeter with clamp-on ammeter

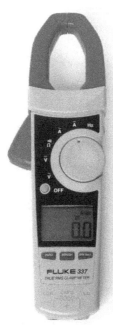

Testing a fuse: Set the meter to read Ω and then touch the black and red to each end of the fuse. If it beeps, then there is continuity and the fuse is good.

Make sure that you do not have the fuse installed or energized when you are doing this test.

HORSEPOWER

Often, pumps and some other electrical equipment are measured in horsepower. It is highly recommended that you know how to convert HP to watts.

1 Horsepower = 746 Watts = 0.746 kW

A 7.5kW system would be about 10 horsepower.

TYPES OF DC CONNECTIONS (SERIES AND PARALLEL)

Often times PV is hooked up in groups of solar modules where the positive lead of one module is connected to the negative lead of the next module. That is called a series connection. With PV and batteries, **series connections increase voltage**.

Even within a solar PV module itself, the solar cells are connected in series to increase voltage.

Parallel connections do not increase voltage and increase only current with PV.

Series: Positive to negative and increases voltage.

Parallel: All of the positives are connected to one place and all of the negatives to another.

With alternating current, we can also have series and parallel connections.

An ac series connection would be like hooking up those Christmas lights that all go out when one goes out. This is analogous to wiring PV in series and when one PV module is shaded, it reduces the current through all of the PV modules (unless a bypass diode kicks in see page 000). In a series connection, if the current goes through one thing, it then goes through whatever it is in series with.

Figure 3.5 Diagram of a PV system, including series and parallel connections

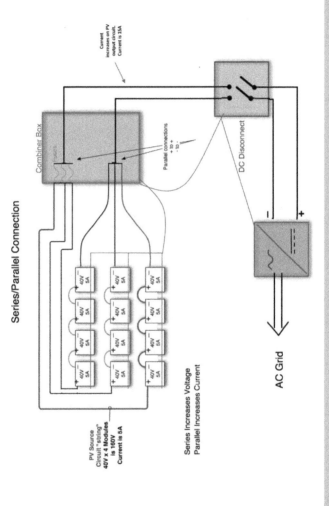

Series/Parallel Connection

Current increases on PV output circuit. Current is 15A

Combiner Box

Parallel connections
+ to +
− to −

DC Disconnect

AC Grid

PV Source Circuit "string" is 160V
40V x 4 Modules
Current is 5A

Series Increases Voltage
Parallel Increases Current

40V 5A

Statistics for an average solar PV module:

- An average solar module is often called a solar panel, but technically it is a solar module.

- An average residential solar module has 60 solar cells connected in series. You can see the connections going from the front of one cell to the back of the next. (Usually the front is the negative side of the cell.)

- An average solar module for a larger job has 72 solar cells connected in series.

- The average solar cell is 6 inches (156 mm) in diameter.

- The average 60 cell solar module is 250 to 300 Watts (0.25kW to 0.3kW).

- The average 72 cell solar module is 300 to 340 Watts.

- As time goes on average solar modules become more efficient.

- The average 60 cell solar module is slightly less than 40 inches wide and slightly less than 66 inches long. That is about 1 meter x 1.67 meter.

- A 72 cell module is about 1 foot longer than a 60 cell module, which is about 1 meter x 2 meters.

- A datasheet with the specifications of a solar module can be easily found by searching "270W solar pdf" on the Internet.

Even with water flow in solar hot water systems, we can have series and parallel connections. As solar PV becomes less expensive, solar hot water systems are less often cost effective.

Ac parallel connections are the connections that are made at a subpanel. Various circuits are connected together with a parallel connection.

ELECTRICAL TRANSMISSION AND DISTRIBUTION SYSTEMS

Most often, electricity is made at huge centralized power plants at high voltages by rotating machinery. Solar is rapidly overtaking other forms of new energy installations.

Figure 3.6 Series and parallel connections. Light bulbs on the right are connected in series to each other. Light bulb in the middle is connected in parallel with the other bulbs

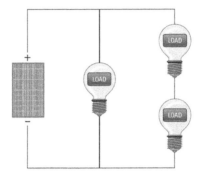

The voltage is stepped up for long distance transmission and then stepped down for our use. High voltage has fewer losses. High voltage is good for transmission, but can cause a big spark (arcing), so is not as good for utilization, which is why we do not have 1000V outlets.

Why we transmit electricity with high voltage:

Voltage × Current = Power

Higher current causes voltage drop and power loss on transmission lines, so if we can transmit our power with high voltage and low current, then we have fewer losses.

A 1kW 12V battery based system would have 4 times more losses than a 1kW 24V battery based system or 16 times the losses of a 1kW 48V system if we were using the same conductors (wires).

When we lose power on a conductor, it is because of "voltage drop". If we measured the voltage of where power is coming from and where it is going to, we would always have more voltage where the power is coming from. In a PV system, the voltage is coming from the PV to the inverter and coming from the inverter to the grid.

Transmitting electricity over long distances and raising and lowering voltages with transformers always leads to losses. A big benefit of PV is that we can make the electricity where we are using it and do not have to have distribution or transformer losses. Making it where we are using it is called Distributed Generation (DG). The fastest growing part of the industry is with large utility scale PV systems, due to economies of scale.

Nikola Tesla first came up with alternating current and transformers. He showed that we could step up and down voltages, so that we can transmit power over long distances with high voltage. Transformers do not work with dc power. To change the current and voltage like a transformer does with direct current, we can use dc-to-dc converters. Often times solar installers are putting dc-to-dc converters at the module level and are calling these dc-to-dc converters "power optimizers".

What is high voltage?

There are many different definitions of high, medium and low voltage. Utilities think of 600V or 1000V and below as low voltage. Laypeople think of 600V as high voltage.

People that work with 12V lighting systems think of 12V as low voltage.

Inverter companies sell medium voltage ready inverters and they are referring to medium voltage as thousands of volts (kV).

Figure 3.7 Electrical generation, transmission and distribution system

Source: Wikimedia Commons. Attribution: J JMesserly https://en.vwikipedia.org/wiki/File:Electricity_grid_simple-_NOrth_America.svg.
This file is licensed under the Creative Commons Attribution 3.0 Unported license.

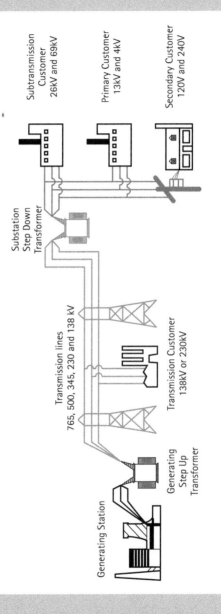

CHAPTER 3 PV MATH (ANSWERS ON PAGE 176)

1. A 200-watt light is left on for 7 days. How much energy is consumed?
   a. 34kWh
   b. 336kW
   c. 3360Wh
   d. 14MWh

2. If a 100W light bulb is working on a 120V socket, what is the current?
   a. 12kW
   b. 0.83A
   c. 1.2A
   d. 144 Ω

3. How much resistance does the light bulb have in question 2 above?
   a. 0.83 ohms
   b. 12 ohms
   c. 0.007 Ω
   d. 144 Ω

4. The hydraulic analogy for voltage is
   a. Flow
   b. Volume
   c. Capacity
   d. Pressure

5. The hydraulic analogy for current is
   a. Flow
   b. Volume
   c. Capacity
   d. Pressure

6. Current required to send one MW (million watts) at the voltage of one MV (million volts)?

    a. 1A

    b. 1 million Amperes

    c. 1Ah

    d. 100A

7. 2000 watts is equal to

    a. 20kW

    b. 2kW

    c. 0.2kW

    d. 2kWh

8. The power of a 250-watt solar module is equal to

    a. 1/4th of a kW

    b. 0.025MW

    c. 25KVA

    d. 0.25kWh

9. One horsepower equals

    a. 0.746kW

    b. 746kWh

    c. 1000W

    d. 1MW

10. A pump works at 4A and 12V for 3 hours. How much energy does it consume?

    a. 144kWh

    b. 48Wh

    c. 0.144kWh

    d. 96Wh

Answers in back of book on page 176.

Solar energy fundamentals

SOLAR POWER

Measured in **power per unit area** and most often in **watts per square meter.**

1000 watts per square meter is called **"peak sun"**, which is a typical sunny day near noon.

SOLAR ENERGY

Since: power × time = energy

Then: **solar power × time = solar energy**

If we have **peak sun conditions of 1000 watts per square meter** for one hour, then we have a **"peak sun hour"** or a **"sun hour"**.

Different locations have different amounts of solar energy. We often quantify the amount of energy a location has in average **peak sun hours per day.**

Peak sun hours per day is also often called insolation. **Insolation is incident solar radiation.**

Table 4.1 gives some insolation data for various locations when the solar collector is tilted at a latitude tilt angle. (Latitude is the angular degrees from the equator, which we will learn more about later in this chapter.)

PSH = Peak Sun Hour = 1kWh/m^2/day at latitude tilt.

Table 4.1 Insolation data (south facing at latitude tilt)

Location	Daily insolation
San Francisco	5.4 PSH
Las Vegas	6.5 PSH
Seattle	3.7 PSH
Honolulu	5.7 PSH
Guam	5.1 PSH
New York City	4.6 PSH
Chicago	4.4 PSH

Insolation data from NREL Redbook, http://rredc.nrel.gov/solar/pubs/redbook/

Standard Test Conditions:

● **1000 watts per square meter**
● **25°C (77°F)**
● **1.5 Atmospheric Mass**

Standard Test Conditions (STC) are **how PV modules are tested** and are the conditions under which the module performance is measured. These are the data, which are put on the label and determine how many watts the module has, which determines the price. Sometimes PV will make more power, current and voltage than what it says on the label (STC) when it is bright and/or cold. Most often, the PV module will make less than it says on the label, since it is usually less bright than 1000W/square meter and it is often hotter than 25°C.

> Four 250W PV modules make 1 kW of PV.
> Forty 250W PV modules make 10kW of PV.
> Four thousand 250W PV modules make 1MW of PV.

Often it is stated as **10kWp** where the p stands for peak sun conditions, which is also STC.

The temperature will determine the voltage. Cooler PV works better and has better voltage. **Lower temperatures increase PV voltage.**

Figure 4.1 The atmosphere filters more light at greater angles (when the sun is lower)

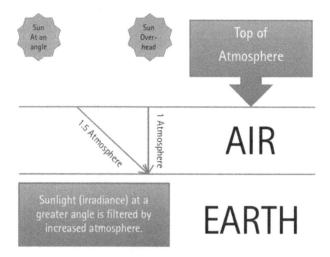

1.5 Atmospheric Mass (AM) is the spectrum of light, which PV is tested in the factory. The test conditions are simulated with a flash of light and a filter to simulate 1.5 AM during PV module testing. The thicker the atmosphere, the less light will make it to the PV. This means that at **higher elevations, sunlight will have less atmosphere to travel through**, which will increase performance (current). Also, around noon and summer solstice, the sun is highest in the sky and will have less atmosphere to travel through, than when the sun is lower in the sky.

The atmosphere is relatively thin compared to the earth. If we painted over a globe, the thickness of the paint would be about that of the atmosphere. If we could drive our car straight up for five minutes at highway speeds, we would reach the edge of the atmosphere. That is not a lot of room to dump 100s of years of CO_2 pollution.

LATITUDE

The equator is zero latitude and the North Pole is 90 degrees latitude. Just like degrees in a compass, the equator is at a 90-degree angle from the North Pole. At **every latitude, the path of the sun is exactly the same all around the world.** Athens Greece and San Francisco California are both at latitude 38 degrees and have the same sun paths. The weather will make solar energy production different however.

SOLAR TIME

In the early 1800s, before there were time zones, we kept time by where the sun was in the sky. **Solar noon** is when the sun is as high in the sky as it will get for the day. In the latitudes of the continental United States and Canada, **solar noon is when the sun is due south.** (In the tropics and Southern Hemisphere, the sun can be north at solar noon.)

As we can see from Figure 4.2, the earth rotates around the sun in the **ecliptic plane.** Most everything in the solar system (and the milky way) rotates around the sun in a similar plane and spins in the same direction.

From a northern hemisphere perspective (where most people are), everything spins counter-clockwise. This is why it is noon in NYC three hours before it is noon in San Francisco.

The earth is tilted about 23.5 degrees; this is what gives us seasons. The equator is facing 23.5 degrees below the sun on summer solstice and is facing 23.5 degrees above the sun on winter solstice.

At equinox, the sun will be right over the equator.

Equinox is Latin for equal nights. At equinox when the sun is right over the equator, the sun will rise at 6am solar time and set at 6pm solar time everywhere in the world (except the north and south poles). Equinox is the only time of the year when the sun rises due east and sets due west. In the northern hemisphere, the sun will rise and set to the north of east and west in the summer and rise and set to the south of due east and west in the winter. At summer solstice at sunrise and sunset, the sun will be more north than south and will shine on a north-facing window.

Figure 4.2 Earth's orbit

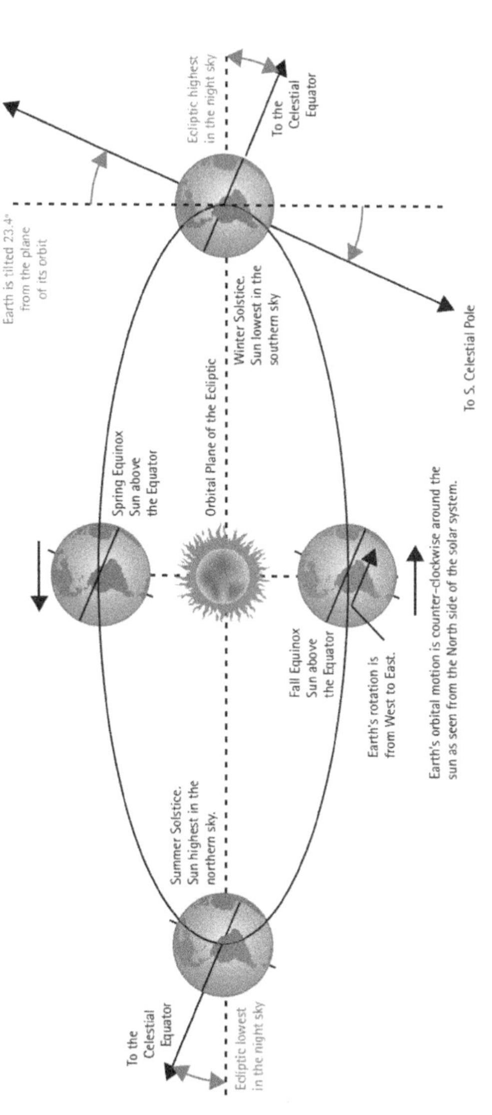

Polaris
To N. Celestial Pole

To the
Celestial
Equator

Ecliptic highest
in the night sky

Earth is tilted 23.4°
from the plane
of its orbit

Winter Solstice.
Sun lowest in the
southern sky

To S. Celestial Pole

Spring Equinox
Sun above
the Equator

Orbital Plane of the Ecliptic

Summer Solstice.
Sun highest in the
northern sky.

Fall Equinox
Sun above
the Equator

Earth's rotation is
from West to East.

Earth's orbital motion is counter-clockwise around the
sun as seen from the North side of the solar system.

To the
Celestial
Equator

Ecliptic lowest
in the night sky

If we want to see the path of the sun plotted on a sun chart, we can do an Internet search for "Oregon Sun Chart" and get a sun chart from the University of Oregon.

By using the sun chart in Figure 4.3, we can predict where the sun will be throughout the year.

On the horizontal x-axis azimuth is plotted.

On the vertical y-axis the elevation of the sun is plotted.

Figure 4.3 Image generated from University of Oregon Sun Chart Program

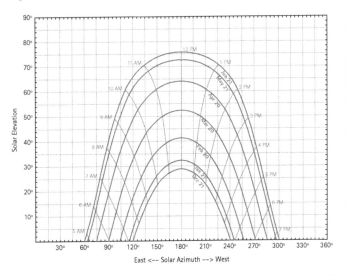

The sun is the highest when it is over the meridian or longitude of where you are located. Meridians or lines of longitude are lines that indicate where a location is in the east and west direction. These lines go from the north to the south poles along the surface of the earth. Meridians or lines of longitude are perpendicular to lines of latitude.

Azimuth is the direction we measure on a compass. North is zero degrees and we go clockwise 360 degrees. East is 90 degrees, south is 180 degrees and west is 270 degrees azimuth.

(Occasionally in the solar industry, we see some systems that use south as zero degrees azimuth.)

Figure 4.4 Azimut altitude.svg

Source: Wikimedia Commons. Attribution: Joshua Cesa. http://commons. wikimedia.org/wiki/File:Azimut_altitude.svg. This file is licensed under the Creative Commons Attribution 3.0 Unported license.

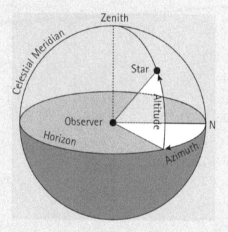

In Figure 4.5, we have a compass with a correction for magnetic declination, such as we see on the West Coast of the United States. The red arrow of the compass is pointing at the magnetic North Pole. The adjustable dial has been rotated counter clockwise towards the geographic North Pole (the axis of the Earth). In the solar industry, we are looking for the path of the sun, which has to do with the axis of the earth. We usually only have to correct for magnetic declination when using a magnetic compass. GPS, maps and many solar devices already correct for magnetic declination. Remember that the magnetic North Pole is over the middle of Canada on the globe.

Figure 4.5 Compass with a correction for magnetic declination
Source: Courtesy of Blake Miller, http://outdoorquest.blogspot.com/2011_09_01_archive.html.

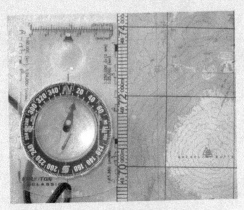

Figure 4.6 Map for correction of magnetic declination

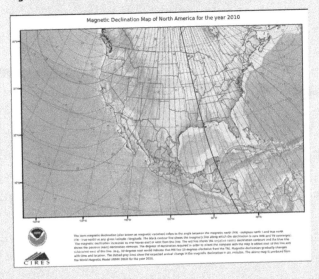

Figure 4.6 shows how we correct for magnetic declination in different locations. For instance, in Florida, we subtract 5 degrees from the azimuth as read on a magnetic compass to correct for magnetic declination.

Figure 4.7 Magnetic North Pole moves slowly
Source: Wikimedia Commons. Attribution: Tentotwo. https://en.wikipedia.org/wiki/File:Magnetic_North_Pole_Positions.svg. This file is licensed under the Creative Commons Attribution-Share Alike 3.0 Unported license.

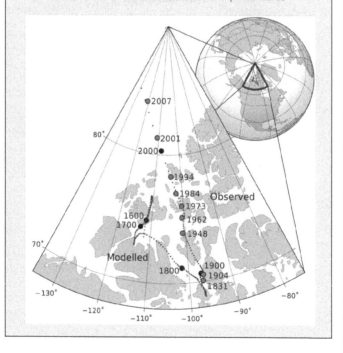

Solar noon by definition is when the sun is highest.

Get to know the sun chart and you can use it to predict shading of a solar array.

You can also be an expert on predicting the best places for sunsets.

If we look more closely at the sun chart, we see that hours are marked with solar noon being when the sun is south. The other hours of the day are also marked. In the months between March and September, the days are longer than the nights and in the months between September and March, the nights are longer than the days.

At equinox, we can see that the sun rises at 6am solar time and sets 12 hours later at 6pm solar time. This is true for all sun charts.

The days closest to the shortest day of the year, which is winter solstice and is approximately December 21, will have the longest shadow.

> The seasons do not always start on the same day throughout the year. This is because of leap years, and the earth's orbit that is not perfectly symmetrical (it is elliptical). Also, in different places on the earth, it is different days at the same time. There is a good chance when you are reading this that it is tomorrow in Asia or yesterday in America.

We can use the sun charts to help determine how much solar energy will be at a certain location and there are devices which can superimpose trees and other objects that cast shadows onto different sun charts.

The two most popular devices are the Solmetric Suneye and the Solar Pathfinder.

With the Solar Pathfinder and the Solmetric Suneye, summer is towards the middle, which corresponds closest to overhead.

On the University of Oregon sun chart, summer is plotted with a higher solar elevation angle over the top.

THE TROPICS

Below 23.5 degrees north latitude, the sun will be directly overhead at times.

The **23.5 degrees north latitude line is called the Tropic of Cancer.**

Above 23.5 degrees south latitude will also have the sun overhead at times and this line is called the **Tropic of Capricorn** (in the southern hemisphere).

Between the Tropic of Cancer and the Tropic of Capricorn is called the tropics. The tropics is the only place where the sun can be overhead.

In the north where the sun never rises at winter solstice nor sets at summer solstice, it is called the arctic and the arctic begins at the **Arctic Circle**, which

Figure 4.8 The Solmetric Suneye is a popular device used for shade analysis and can predict the path of the sun throughout the year.
Source: www.solmetric.com

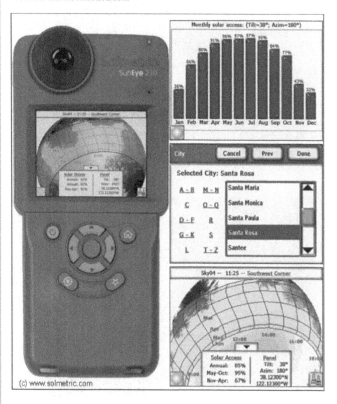

Figure 4.9a and b The Solar Pathfinder is another popular device used to predict shading and the path of the sun throughout the year.
Source: www.solarpathfinder.com

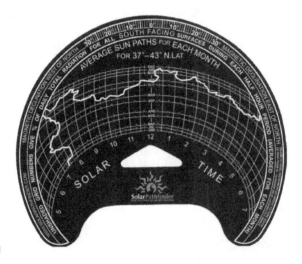

(a)

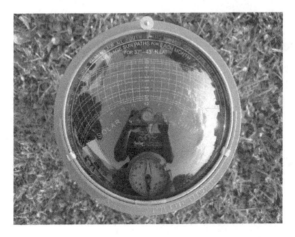

(b)

is at 66.5 degrees latitude. This has to do with the tilt of the earth, which is 23.5 degrees latitude (90°−23.5°=66.5°).

The same can be said for the **Antarctic Circle**, which is at 66.5 degrees south latitude.

Figure 4.10 and 4.11 Angles of the sunlight hitting the earth at winter solstice and summer solstice. By looking at these images, we can see how the sunrays hit the earth at different times of the year.
Source: www.solarpathfinder.com

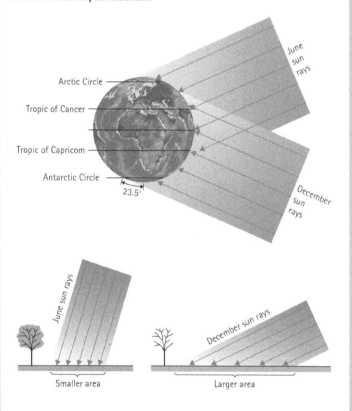

Figure 4.12 The sun paths as viewed from the earth. This is what the sun path looks like in areas that are not in the tropics or the arctic, which is most of the United States and Canada. In the tropics, the sun will be overhead sometimes and in the arctic, it will not rise in the dark of winter.

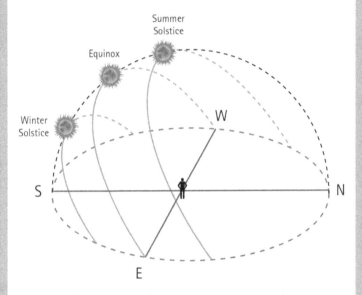

TILT ANGLES

> The sun constantly is moving throughout the sky from our perspectives. It will go 360 degrees in 24 hours, which is 15 degrees per hour and 1 degree every 4 minutes.

When the sun is on the horizon, the elevation angle would be zero degrees. In order for PV to directly face the sun, the PV would have to have a tilt angle of 90 degrees when the sun is on the horizon.

If the sun would be overhead, the optimal tilt angle would be zero degrees.

Tilt of PV is most often based on degrees from the horizontal. Flat is zero tilt and vertical is 90 degrees tilt.

In order to maximize energy production some in the industry would have a tracker that would follow the sun. A **dual axis tracker should always face the sun** and get maximum energy and a **single axis tracker will track the sun on one axis.**

Concentrating PV systems need to use 2-axis trackers to focus direct beam solar radiation, with rare exceptions.

Figure 4.13 A horizontal single axis tracker faces east in the morning and west in the afternoon (flat at solar noon).
Source: Wikimedia Commons. Attribution: Msrt10. http://en.wikipedia.org/wiki/File:RayTracker_Utility_Scale_Solar_Tracker_Installation.JPG. This file is licensed under the Creative Commons Attribution-Share Alike 3.0 Unported license.

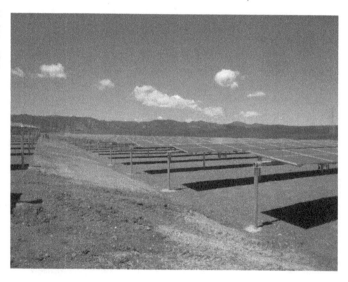

Figure 4.14 2-axis tracker with concentrating PV always faces the sun (Tesla Roadster EV charging)
Source: Wikimedia Commons. Attribution: Mbudzi. http://commons.wikimedia.org/wiki/File:Amonix7700.jpg. This file is licensed under the Creative Commons Attribution-Share Alike 3.0 Unported license.

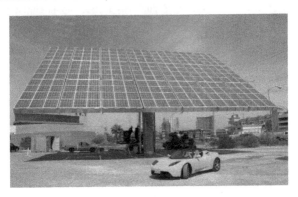

Most often, trackers are not used since they add moving parts and complexity. Depending on where you are and the type of tracker, a tracker can harvest 20–30% more energy than a system without a tracker. As the price of PV drops, trackers are used less. **The exception is with large utility scale PV systems**, where we often have single axis horizontal axis trackers. These trackers face east in the morning, west in the afternoon and are flat at noon. These systems can have a single motor moving hundreds of kW of PV.

Usually on a residential roof, PV is flush mounted to the roof and is put a few inches above the roof facing exactly the way the roof faces.

The US government sponsored National Renewable Energy Laboratory (NREL) has a website that will help you determine energy production. The popular Internet tool is called PV Watts. Do an Internet search for PV Watts for simple PV system production modeling. NREL has many resources for renewable energy education and research. When designing a PV system, it is very important to know how much energy your system will make.

There are many other types of PV simulation software and software is getting better at shade modeling using data from satellites and laser drones (LIDAR). There are good solar jobs opportunities for someone who is good at operating software that can model performance and make sales proposals.

Figure 4.15 Tilt angle optimization for different seasons

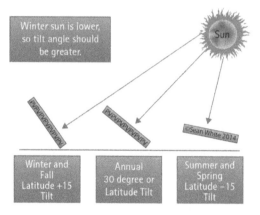

We usually try to get the solar modules facing the direction where they will collect the most energy. There are some "rules of thumb" that we use in the solar industry. They are not exact, but are good to know (often in exams).

Solar rules of thumb:

1. Keep your PV array shade free from 9am to 3pm.
2. Optimize for **summer and spring** production with a tilt of **latitude minus 15 degrees**.
3. Best for **winter and fall** production tilt of **latitude plus 15 degrees**.
4. **Best for annual** production is either latitude tilt or **30-degree** tilt depending on the location.

SHADING

Shading of a PV system is to be avoided, especially when the sun is high in the sky.

Since solar is often wired in series, shading one solar cell can affect the other cells that it is wired in series with. This is often compared to the Christmas light effect: when one light is removed, it will affect the other lights it is wired in series with.

INTER-ROW SHADING

When PV is arranged in multiple rows, the row to the south can shade the row to the north. There are many factors that will help determine how far the rows are to be spaced. The tilt angle, the size of the PV and the height of the back of one row of PV compared to the front of the next row along with the latitude will determine inter-row spacing.

Notice the shadow on the row of modules to the left (Figure 4.16). This is unacceptable unless it is early or late in the day.

In lower latitudes, such as in Miami Florida, rows can be spaced closer together than in places that are farther north, such as in Toronto Canada. This is because places that are farther from the equator have a sun path that is lower in the sky, especially in winter.

Figure 4.17 demonstrates the height of the row and the distance from the back of one row to the front of the next. Often times we talk about a ratio of height to distance of the shading object and the distance away from that object. Closer to the tropics, 2:1 distance:height is acceptable and farther north 3:1 is more acceptable.

Some people use trigonometry (the relationships of triangles) to determine the best inter-row spacing.

Many times, commercial rooftop systems have a lower tilt angle in order to decrease the height of the rows and fit more PV on the roof. Also lowering the tilt will cause less wind uplift forces.

Figure 4.16 M&M candy factory in NJ
Source: Photo by Sean White

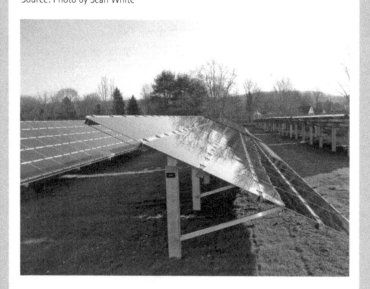

Figure 4.17 Inter-row shading
Source: Image by Sean White

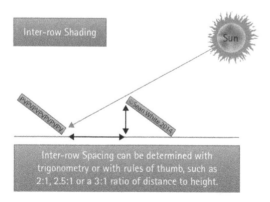

TYPES OF SOLAR RADIATION

Direct: Radiation that comes directly from the sun. The rays of sunlight are parallel to each other.

Diffuse: Radiation that comes from bouncing off of clouds and the atmosphere. The blue sky is an example of diffuse radiation.

Albedo: Radiation that is **reflected** off something else, such as the ground, a white roof, a tree or a lake.

Global: Combined solar radiation from all types.

> Concentrated PV is solar energy, which is captured with lenses or mirrors that focus sunbeams onto solar cells. Concentrated solar only works with direct sunlight and does not work at all on a cloudy day. Concentrated PV only works with a tracker and most often it is a 2-axis tracker that can point the PV at the sun at all times. If you have ever played with a magnifying glass in the sun, you have concentrated sunlight.

WAYS TO MEASURE SOLAR RADIATION

Pyranometer: A device that measures global solar radiation. Also called an irradiance meter. Pyro = fire and meter = measure.

Pyranoheliometer: Measures **direct beam** solar radiation. Direct beam solar radiation is important for concentrating systems.

The sun is constantly moving throughout the sky and weather patterns in the atmosphere make solar energy analysis a science that can be as variable as the weather on a daily basis and as variable as the changing climate on an annual basis.

Most residential rooftop PV systems are not oriented in the perfect direction, but they do produce enough solar energy to be cost effective. As solar systems go down in price, new rooftop space that was not cost effective in the past becomes cost effective. In places like Hawaii where energy is expensive and sunshine is high in the sky, even north facing arrays are now becoming good investments.

I just put solar on my north roof in California. I will make one-third less energy per kW installed on the north roof than I do with the PV on my south roof, however the PV on my north roof was a better investment, since when I installed the PV on the north roof, it was after the price of the PV system was half of what the price was 5 years ago when I installed PV on the south roof. Five years ago, if I told people I installed PV on my north roof, I would have been laughed off the roof! North-facing PV is not always cost effective; it depends on different factors, such as location, utility rates, government incentives and if you install your own system.

You can try simulating the different slopes of your roof at www.pvwatts.nrel.gov. See how differently your north and south facing rooftops will produce energy.

PV module fundamentals

Chapter 5

Albert Einstein won the Nobel Peace Prize for describing the process by which
light interacts with matter and "sets electrons free". He was in the solar
industry, just like you, which is smart.

HOW PV WORKS

Light (photons) hits a semiconductor, increases the energy of electrons and
creates current, voltage and power.

Figure 5.1 P-N junction of a photovoltaic cell
Source: Sean White

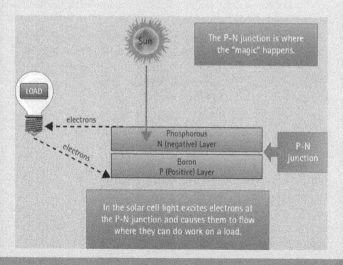

Figure 5.2 Monocrystalline solar cells, rounded corners
Source: Courtesy Suntech

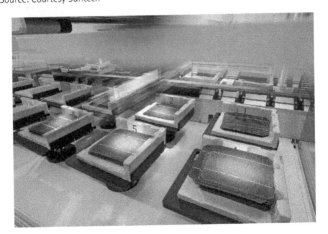

Pure silicon is refined from sand or quartz, and then formed into a large crystal ingot, which is then sliced into thin wafers. Wafers are then prepared by adding different layers of phosphorous, anti-reflective coatings and screen-printed silver contacts for catching electrons. There are different variations on this theme, but this is your typical process.

Nominal Voltage: Nominal means "in name only". The nominal voltage of your car battery is 12V (2 volts per battery cell). The nominal voltage of a silicon solar cell is one third of a volt. 36 cell PV modules were popular in the past, because they were 12V nominal (36 × one third = 12V). Before grid-tied solar was popular, we would match PV voltage to battery voltage at a ratio of 6 PV cells to each lead acid battery cell.

PV, batteries and your house rarely work at "nominal" voltage. Your car battery is over 14V when you are driving and your solar cell voltage fluctuates depending on the temperature, what the cell is connected to and if the solar cell is turned on or off.

Solar cells are combined to create a solar module. An average solar module consists of 60 or 72 solar cells connected together in series.

Figure 5.3 Polycrystalline/multicrystalline solar module
Source: Courtesy Yingli Solar

> Multicrystalline solar cells are cast cells with square corners. Most solar cells produced are multicrystalline (polycrystalline).

Monocrystalline is typically more efficient than polycrystalline solar; however the differences are not usually very significant, especially since monocrystalline is usually more expensive and has a higher carbon footprint.

The **most efficient solar cells** are made from a material called **Gallium Arsenide**. This is very expensive and usually used for outer space and concentrating PV applications.

Other types of thin film solar are

1. Cadmium Telluride
2. CIGS Copper Indium Gallium Selenide
3. Amorphous Silicon.

Thin film is not as popular, because it is typically not as efficient and cost effective as crystalline silicon PV.

SOLAR PANEL

Most people call a solar module a solar panel.

Figure 5.4 Solar panel made from solar modules
Source: Courtesy Sunlink

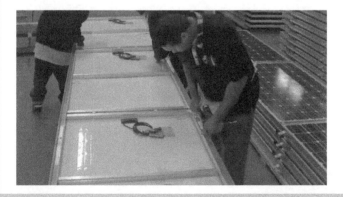

Figure 5.5 A PV array is a larger group of modules.
Source: Wikimedia Commons. https://commons.wikimedia.Org/wiki/File:Vermont_
Law_Sehool_Solar_Panel_Array-1.JPG. This file is made available under the Creative
Commons CCO 1.0 Universal Public Domain Dedication.

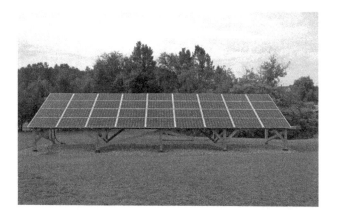

Technically, a **solar panel is a group of modules** preconfigured as a unit before
they are installed.

CALCULATING EFFICIENCY OF A SOLAR MODULE

Efficiency is the ratio of watts per square meter of output at STC to the irradiance at STC, which is 1000 watts per square meter.

For instance, if a PV module was making 150 watts per square meter, then 150
watts per square meter output /1000 watts per square meter (STC) input = 0.15
or 15% efficiency.

Let us do an example calculation:

Example 250W PV Module
Dimensions 1638 × 982mm

1.638m × 0.982m = 1.6 square meters
250W/1.6 square meters = 156W/square meter

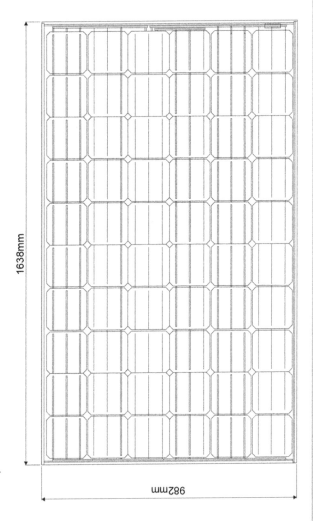

Figure 5.6 Typical solar module dimensions in mm

Source: Courtesy Canadian Solar

1638mm

982mm

STC is 1000 watts per square meter
156W/1000W = 0.156
0.156 × 1000/0 = 15.6% efficient PV

ESTIMATING HOW MUCH PV FITS IN A GIVEN SPACE

If you covered 100 square meters with 15.6% efficient PV, you would have

156W/square meter × 100 square meters
15,600W = 15.6kW of PV

In reality, you would need extra space around the edges and chimneys, since you usually cannot fit PV in every space.

Some designers estimate 100W to 150W/square meter, to leave room for roof penetrations, walkways and space for firefighters. Making a quick estimate can get you in the ballpark. If you are American, you might want to estimate that you can install about 100 to 150W per square foot.

Do not use dissimilar PV modules in series.

When PV is connected in series, you will have what is sometimes called "the Christmas light effect". **If one module has less current, then it will limit the amount of current to flow through the whole series connected PV source circuit (string).**

Before there were bypass diodes in PV modules, when a cell was shaded all of the current from all of the other cells and modules would try to push through

Figure 5.7 Module mismatch

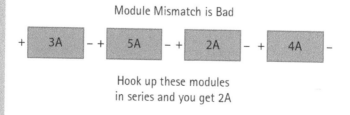

Module Mismatch is Bad

Hook up these modules
in series and you get 2A

Figure 5.8 PV module with bypass diodes
Source: Courtesy of Solmetric

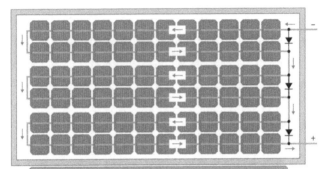

Shading of the long edge is more desirable than shading of
the short edge due to the arrangement of the diodes.
Shading a row on the short edge will take out all 3 sections.

the shaded cell. This would create heat (from resistance) and could be a fire hazard. Also, it would be terrible for performance.

This is similar to what happens with shading or different orientations within a string.

Bypass diodes will bypass a group of cells. The group of cells being bypassed would not create voltage, but would let the current through. Most PV modules have three bypass diodes, separating the module into three separate sections. If a shadow would cover a cell or a number of cells in a group, the bypass diode would bypass the entire third of the module. 60-cell modules have cells arranged 6 x 10 and have 20 cells per bypass diode and 72-cell modules have cells arranged 6 x 12 with 24 cells per bypass diode.

Bypass diodes sacrifice voltage for current.

A bypass diodes analogy would be: When there is an accident on the freeway, you take the side streets.

Bypass diodes are **wired in parallel** to a group of cells so there is another (parallel) pathway for current to take when there is a shaded cell.

Bypass diodes help mitigate the holiday light effect of shading interfering with the stoppage of current. Someone selling a technology where modules are not connected in series with each other, such as with a microinverter or a dc-to-dc converter (see page 83), may have a tendency to overstate the series losses and forget about the bypass diodes when comparing their technology to PV circuits that have many PV modules connected in series.

BLOCKING DIODES

Blocking diodes are not used in the typical PV system these days, however in the past they were popular. They **prevent reverse current**. In plumbing an analogy would be a check valve. Another highway analogy is a one-way street.

Blocking diodes are wired in series. (Bypass diodes are parallel connected.)

IV CURVES (I = CURRENT AND V = VOLTAGE)

(Good section to bookmark and review)

Voc = OPEN CIRCUIT VOLTAGE

In Figure 5.9 we can see the point called Voc (open circuit voltage). Voc is the point at which there is an open circuit. This means that the **PV system is turned off**. As we can see, the voltage is as high as it can get, but the current is zero. Since voltage multiplied by current is power, then:

Voc × Zero Amps = Zero power (Amps is current is I)

It is interesting that when you turn off a PV system, the voltage will increase. That means you can still get shocked when PV is off.

ISC = SHORT CIRCUIT CURRENT

Short circuit current (Isc) is the upper left point on the IV curve where there is **all current and no voltage**. This is an operating point that hopefully your PV system will never experience. A short happens when there is a **direct** connection

Figure 5.9 I-V curve
Source: Courtesy Solmetric

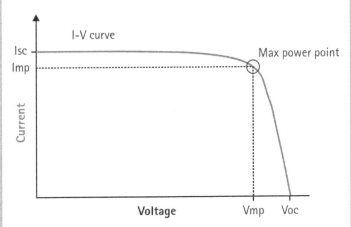

between positive and negative. This is the point of the most current, where voltage is zero. Once again anything multiplied by zero is zero, so Isc is not a power-producing situation.

Isc × Zero Volts = Zero Power

If conductors are installed incorrectly and the insulation of the wire disappears or is damaged, you can have a positive to negative short. This can cause a fuse in a dc combiner box to blow. Dc combiners are less common in PV systems on buildings than they used to be and are most often seen with large utility scale systems when there are inverters that are often a MW.

Vmp = MAXIMUM POWER VOLTAGE

At maximum power voltage, we have the point of maximum power. This means that we want to operate in this position to get the most out of our PV. It is interesting to note that "maximum" power voltage is less than open circuit voltage. It is not the maximum voltage, it is the voltage at maximum power.

Imp = MAXIMUM POWER CURRENT

Imp is maximum power current and this is at the same point as Vmp.

If we multiply Imp × Vmp we will get the maximum power at the maximum power point.

Maximum power current is less than short circuit current.

Vmp × Imp = Maximum Power = Power of the PV module

For example, if we have a PV module where the Vmp is 30 Volts and the Imp is 8 Amps then:

30 Vmp × 8 Amp = 240W

We have a 240W PV module

Often students get confused and think that Vmp or Imp is the higher voltage or current, since **m** is for maximum, however it is not the case. Isc is higher current than Imp, but at Isc there is no power, not maximum power. Isc is not a power-producing place, and the same goes for Voc.

Another common **mistake** people make is **multiplying Voc and Isc** and getting some imaginary power. This does not get you power!

If we look at Isc at the upper left part of the IV curve, and see how the line gradually slopes down to the maximum power point (MPP) we see places where power is made, but not as much as the power made at the MPP. It is interesting that **at the point of the most current, there is no power at all.**

Most inverters can keep the PV working at the MPP and we call this maximum power point tracking or **MPPT**.

Summary:

Voc × Zero Amps = Zero Power
Isc × Zero Volts = Zero Power
Vmp × Imp = Maximum Power
Voc × Isc: PV cannot operate here

FACTORS THAT CHANGE PERFORMANCE OF PV

When PV is made and sold it is rated at STC (Standard Test Conditions)

STC
1000W/m²   (brightness of light about like noon)
25°C   (77°F)
1.5AM   (Air Mass spectrum of light)

We need to be able to compare PV modules and determine which is the best deal. When we pay a per watt price, we are getting the PV rated at STC.

In the real world, PV operates under different conditions.

The **best production we can get is on a bright cold day**. Mt. Everest may be a good place for PV!

TEMPERATURE AND VOLTAGE (ENVIRONMENTAL CONDITIONS)

Figure 5.10 Temperature and irradiance effects on voltage and current
Source: Sean White

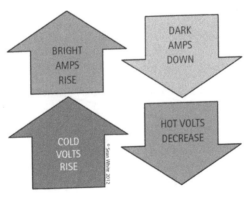

BRIGHT = MORE CURRENT

Brightness means more light (photons) knocking electrons loose, which translates to more current (amps). We call bright light increased irradiance and since **irradiance starts with the letter I**, then it is easy to remember that it increases I (symbol for **current**).

COLD = MORE VOLTAGE

Cold temperatures increase voltage. Some students think of the T in vol**t** to remember.

Silicon semiconductors just work better in the cold. That is why your computer has a fan that cools the silicon computer chip.

The problem with cold temperatures increasing voltage is that sunlight, which is good for solar cells, causes heat, which is bad for power production. It is a good enough trade off though and many solar modules are installed in the hottest deserts. The increased sunlight makes up for the loss of voltage due to heat.

On the left of Figure 5.11 are IV curves with different amounts of irradiance (light) with a constant temperature. We can see how **more irradiance increases I (current)**.

On the image on the right of Figure 5.11, we can see that when the temperature is changed voltage changes. **Colder temperatures cause higher voltages**. That is why we like to mount our PV so that there is **airflow, to blow the heat away**.

PV can get very hot in the sun. But it is better to have a hot sunny day than a cold dark day, because with darkness, you lose more power than with heat.

In Figure 5.12, we can see how PV stacks up with series and parallel connections.

This image represents **two strings (PV source circuits) of three modules in series**.

Figure 5.15 lets us see how voltage increases with series connections. On a cold day, this voltage will increase even more.

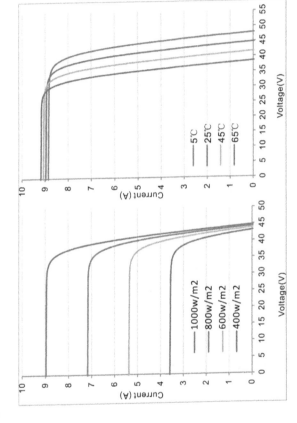

Figure 5.11 Irradiance and temperature effects on I–V curves
Source: Courtesy Canadian Solar

Figure 5.12 I-V curve representation 2 PV source circuits (strings) of 3 in series

Source: Courtesy of Solmetric

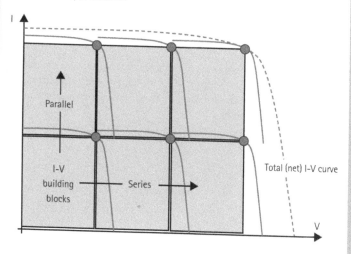

DIFFERENT WAYS OF TESTING PV

Table 5.1 PV testing conditions

STC	NOCT	CEC	PTC
25°C cell	20°C ambient	20°C ambient	20°C ambient
1000W/m²	800W/m²	1000W/m²	1000W/m²
	1m/sec wind	1m/sec wind	1m/sec wind

STC (Standard Test Conditions) is measured in watts and is the standard way modules are tested and sold. STC is what is always indicated on the back of the module. Note that STC does not have an airspeed as do the rest of the testing conditions. This is because STC is tested at cell temperature rather than ambient temperature.

NOCT (Nominal Operating Cell Temperature) is the temperature that the PV solar cell heats up to when exposed to NOCT test conditions.

CEC (California Energy Commission) and **PTC** (Performance Test Conditions) are similar derived, which are extrapolated with different formulae. This is a lower power than STC because of the solar cells heating up usually about 30°C above ambient temperature in the sunlight.

AM (Air Mass) 1.5

All of the tests are carried out with the spectrum of light equivalent to **1.5 air mass**. By definition 1 air mass is when the sun is directly overhead at sea level. This test was standardized when the atmosphere was measured at Cape Canaveral Florida on Equinox.

PV module label data requirements:

1. **STC Watts**
2. **Voc**
3. **Vmp**
4. **Imp**
5. **Isc**
6. **Maximum series fuse rating**
7. **STC conditions**

Not required on PV label:

1. CEC (California Energy Commission)
2. NOCT (Nominal Operating Cell Temperature)
3. Minimum fuse rating (no such thing).

Explanations:

Maximum series fuse rating is on the PV module, because if you had a fuse that was too big (too much current before opening the circuit) then it would not protect the module assembly. We say the module assembly includes the connectors and everything else that comes with the module. Most modules have a 15A or 20A max series fuse rating. If you put a 30A fuse on it, then it would not protect the module and that would be a safety issue. If you put a 5A fuse on it, it would protect it, but you would have blown fuses opening circuits when you did not need to, which is not a safety issue.

PV AS A LIMITED CURRENT SOURCE

PV Isc is only about 7% more than Imp. Usually when electricians are working with conventional electricity, they have a current source that can be much greater than the operating current. There are benefits and drawbacks to this.

When we pull current out of the wall in our house, there is a constant voltage source and we take as much current as we need. When there is a short, too much current causes a circuit breaker or fuse, aka, Over Current Protection Device (OCPD) to turn the system off by opening the circuit.

With PV, since the short circuit current is not much more than maximum power current a fuse will not always open the circuit when there is a short. This is the drawback.

A benefit is that there is not too much extra available current unlike with conventional power.

"Listed" PV modules must be used in the United States, Canada and most of the developed world. The PV modules in North America must be listed to the **UL Standard 1703**. This means that there are standards developed by UL and that a testing laboratory must test the PV to that standard. (UL 1741 is for inverters.) Europeans typically look for the CE listing of the PV module and some countries will accept either.

When PV is used to charge batteries **without** an MPPT charge controller, the PV voltage will have to match the battery voltage. 36 PV cells will work best for charging a 12V battery at about 14.5 volts.

System components (definitions)

SYSTEM COMPONENTS

PV module: Turns light into electricity. A group of solar cells in a sealed unit.

Interactive inverter: Often called **grid-tied inverter**. An inverter that reads the voltage of the grid or microgrid and produces as much power and current as it can, regardless of loads. For instance, a 5kW inverter can only put out 5kW. Grid tied inverters are sold according to maximum output power. They also have dc and ac operating voltage ranges.

Microinverter: A small inverter that is mounted behind a PV module.

String inverter: An inverter that has PV source circuits (modules connected in series, aka, strings) connected to the inverter.

Central inverter: A large inverter, usually in the MW (1000 kW) range without PV source circuits connected directly to the inverter. The PV source circuits are connected together in the field in dc combiners and PV output circuits come out of the combiners to the inverter.

AC module: A module with ac output listed for such use. Can be a microinverter mounted on a module if it was tested together.

Dc-to-dc converter (power optimizer): Often mounted behind modules and convert voltage and current. Can often perform other tasks, such as monitoring and turning of PV modules. Transformers do for ac what dc-to-dc converters do for dc.

Loads: Devices that use energy. A lightbulb is a load.

Conductors: Wires.

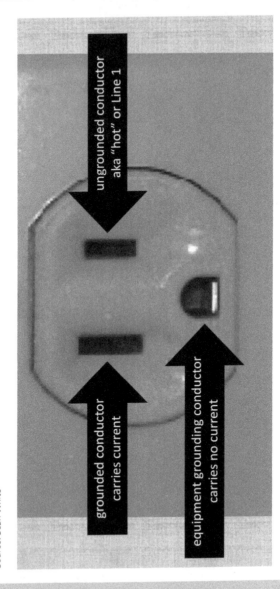

Figure 6.1 North American plug. Grounded conductor and ground at zero volts relative to 120V at ungrounded conductor.
Source: Sean White

Conductor sizes: From small (larger numbers) to larger (smaller numbers). 18AWG is a small wire, 1/0AWG is a large wire and 4/0 (0000) is larger than 1/0. In order of increasing size wire sizes commonly used from **small to large** are **18AWG, 16AWG, 14AWG, 12AWG, 10AWG, 12AWG, 10AWG, 8AWG, 6AWG, 4AWG, 2AWG, 1AWG, 1/0AWG, 2/0AWG, 3/0AWG, 4/0AWG**. Most of the world uses cross-sectional area of wire in square mm for wire sizes.

AWG: American Wire Gauge.

Grounded conductor: A conductor that is intentionally referenced to ground, but carries current. The color of the grounded conductor is **white (or gray)**. In ac wiring the grounded conductor is also called a neutral. Many PV systems installed in the past in the US were negatively grounded where negative was white, while the ungrounded positive was usually black. This is not a typo: **the black wire on a negatively grounded PV system was positive and the white wire was negative**. The black wire can also be red to avoid confusion. The rule is that the grounded conductor must be white or gray. If you are doing maintenance on older PV systems, you will see white negatives and black positives.

Changes in the NEC – functional grounded inverters

Once the 2017 National Electric Code was enforced, a white dc wire on an inverter became extremely rare with new installations. The new naming system changed our descriptions of inverters. If you see literature talking about grounded inverters and ungrounded inverters, chances are that you are referring to 2014 NEC naming systems. Grounded and ungrounded inverters after the 2017 NEC are as rare as unicorns. 99% of interactive inverters installed since 2000 are called Functional Grounded inverters according to the 2017 NEC and beyond. Usually NEC changes do not affect the material covered on the NABCEP Associate exam.

Grounding conductor (equipment grounding conductor or EGC): A conductor that is not meant to carry current and connects (bonds) metal equipment together, so that there are no dangerous voltage differences. A grounding conductor is **green or a bare** wire. Often people remember that a grounding

Figure 6.2 Grid-tied system components

Grid tied system components DC wiring

PV Source Circuit(s) — PV source circuit conductors — Combiner Box — PV output circuit conductors — DC disconnect — inverter input circuit conductors — Inverter — inverter output circuit conductors — AC disconnect

*ac disconnect is often backfed circuit breaker. AC wiring unique to various connection point locations.

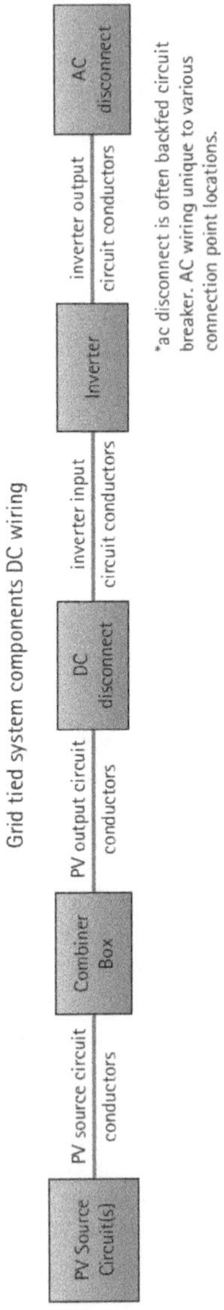

conductor is green or bare, because "grounding" ends with the letter G. Even **"ungrounded systems" have equipment grounding**.

Load center: A place where loads are connected, such as a panelboard, also known as a main service panel (MSP) or a subpanel.

Branch circuit: A circuit coming from a circuit breaker off of a load center. Inverters have dedicated branch circuits.

Transformer: A device used for changing one ac voltage to another ac voltage.

Non-isolated inverter: An inverter without a transformer. Formerly known as an **ungrounded inverter**. Also known as a transformerless inverter (TL). This inverter does not have a current carrying conductor that is at the same voltage as ground. This is the most popular inverter in the world and is very safe. This is a type of **functional grounded inverter**.

PV source circuits (strings): PV modules connected together in series including the PV modules and the conductors. **Voltage increases in series** connected PV source circuits and **current does NOT increase as a result of series connections**.

String sizing: Determining the number of PV modules to be connected in series so that voltage is not too high when it is **cold (causes higher voltage)** and voltage is not too low on hot days (under voltage).

PV source circuit conductors: Connects the PV to the inverter or dc combiner. Unless there is a large inverter, a **dc combiner is often NOT used** and PV source circuits often go to the inverter. If there is just one string, there is no need for a dc combiner (nothing to combine) and the PV source circuit conductors will connect the PV to the inverter.

USE-2 wire and PV wire: Common wiring method for PV source circuits where conductors are exposed to sunlight or not protected in conduit. Can be used exposed or in "free air". PV wire is better and more expensive than USE-2 wire.

Conduit: Pipe that is used for protecting wires.

Raceway: A place where wires are protected. Conduit is a type of a raceway.

Dc combiner: Also known as a combiner box. Where **PV source circuits are combined to become a PV output circuit**. Combiner boxes usually contain fuses when three or more PV source circuits are combined. Combiner boxes are **where parallel connections are made. Parallel connections increase current and do NOT increase voltage**. A blown fuse in a combiner can mean a positive to negative short in a PV source circuit. Dc combiners are most often used with larger inverters such as 1MW (1000kW) utility scale inverters.

Junction box: An electrical box where connections are made.

PV output circuit: At the output of a dc combiner is the PV output circuit. The current of the PV output circuit is the combined current of the PV source circuits (strings) going into the dc combiner.

Ground fault protection device: Interactive (grid-tied) inverters always contain **dc ground fault protection**.

DC disconnect: A switch that **disconnects (opens the circuit)** of dc conductors. DC disconnects are most often found in or near the inverter and near dc combiners. **PV dc disconnects are not allowed in bathrooms**.

AC disconnect: A switch that disconnects (turns off) ac circuit conductors. A circuit breaker is a disconnect and also an over current protection device.

Over Current Protection Device (OCPD): Protects equipment and conductors from over currents. OCPDs will open the circuit if the current gets high enough. PV module source circuits in combiner boxes are usually protected by 15A or 20A fuses, which is the typical PV **maximum series fuse rating**. The two types of OCPDs are fuses or circuit breakers.

Circuit breaker: An OCPD and a disconnect all in one.

Service panel: Also called **panelboard** or **load center**. Where circuit breakers are connected to the electrical system. The main service panel is the main one in the building. Other **sub-panels are connected to the main panel via feeders**. Breakers are connected on busbars.

Busbar: A piece of metal where different circuits are connected in parallel. Usually where breakers or wires are connected.

OFF-GRID SPECIFIC SYSTEM COMPONENTS

Battery: Stores energy by chemical reactions. Many stand-alone PV systems use lead acid batteries.

Flooded lead acid battery: A battery that has a liquid electrolyte (fluid) and uses chemical reactions between lead and acid to store energy.

Sealed valve regulated flooded lead acid battery: A battery that is often called maintenance free, since **you cannot add fluids to a sealed battery**. The valves are for releasing gasses, so the battery does not explode.

Lithium batteries: Often installed in an energy storage system, which includes electronics and is not maintained in the field.

Charge controller: Controller that regulates charging of batteries, **so they are not overcharged or undercharged**. Controllers can be for stand-alone systems or grid-tied battery backup systems. The **highest voltage** for a charge controller is for the **equalization charge**, which is only used on flooded lead acid batteries that fluid can be added to. The equalization charge is for battery maintenance and only done on flooded lead acid batteries that are **not sealed**.

Flow battery: Battery similar to fuel cell where electrolytes are pumped between reactor and storage tanks.

Battery inverter: An inverter that gets voltage from a battery and produces current and power, as it is needed. A battery inverter is hooked up to a battery (often via a charge controller) and not to the PV.

Battery inverter input circuit: The conductors between the battery and the battery inverter, which are **sized according to** the power of the inverter and the **lowest battery voltage**. A lower voltage requires more current for the same power since **power = voltage × current**.

Dc coupled system: A typical off-grid system where charge controllers are used to charge batteries.

Ac coupled system: A system where **interactive inverters** (grid tied) are used with **battery inverters** to charge batteries.

Grid-tied battery-backup system: A system that **works with or without the utility**. Inverters that can operate in both modes are called **bimodal** or **multi-modal inverters**.

Maximum Power Point Tracking (MPPT) charge controllers: Grid-tied inverters are MPPT and many charge controllers are MPPT. MPPT is only for devices that are connected to PV and will optimize production. MPPT controls the IV parameters and will **cause the inverter or charge controller to work on the point of maximum power on the IV curve**. An off-grid inverter connected to a battery does not have MPPT.

PV system sizing principles

Chapter 7

To size a PV system, one must know how much sunlight comes into the system and how much energy is needed to come out of the system, taking into consideration the price of the system.

There are many ways to size PV systems, but the big differences are between grid-tied utility interactive and stand-alone off-grid systems.

Stand-alone systems are made to work alone and will have to be sized so that they work during the worst conditions of the year, which usually means getting through a dark December. The month with the worst solar irradiation we call the **critical design month**. In the summer time, there is usually extra energy that could have been used, but is not produced, because it is not needed in an off-grid system. Also, stand-alone systems have extra energy loss due to inefficiencies with charging and discharging batteries.

With a **grid-tied system**, in almost all situations, every ac kWh (unit of energy) is used and if the customer is not using the energy onsite, it can be exported to the grid so that others may use the energy. With net-metering, the producer of the electricity will get credit for exported energy and be able to use it months later.

There are always customers who ask to use batteries and be independent from the grid, when they are connected to the grid. Financially, this is not a good investment. Batteries are expensive and customers will not be able to export energy and get credit for it later.

Some customers want to have battery backed up systems when they are connected to the grid. This has not been a common practice, because it is a complicated and expensive installation that most PV installers try to discourage their customers from implementing.

Batteries are getting more popular however with the advent of solar PV taking over the world! Since solar and wind are intermittent resources, it makes sense to store the energy on a grid scale or at your home. Additionally, as more solar penetrates the grid, the utilities are more likely to limit the amount someone can export or to decrease the amount of credit someone will get from sending energy back to the grid. In some places with a lot of solar penetration, such as some neighborhoods in Hawaii, customers are not allowed to export any energy to the grid. They can still be connected to the grid, but when they are using less than they are producing, they either have to send the extra energy to a battery or slow down their interactive inverter.

Some systems with batteries do not have the ability to work when the grid is not functioning. The batteries take the extra energy from the day and will supplement the usage at night. This is called **self-consumption** by many in the industry. These self-consumption inverter/battery systems often do have the ability to have backup power, but not always.

BASIC SYSTEM SIZING FACTORS

Grid tied system sizing (without batteries):

1. Space available for system
2. Energy production goal in kWh/yr
3. Customer budget
4. Incentives.

Off-grid system sizing:

1. Energy requirements
2. Power requirements
3. Reducing loads (efficiency)
4. Battery budget
5. PV budget
6. Days of autonomy

Regardless if the system is utility interactive or stand-alone, the location derating factors also are a factor in determining system size.

To simplify system sizing, we can look to this basic grid tied example and from there:

AC kW system size x derating x insolation = production

Example: PV system produces **4kW** at 1000W per square meter of irradiation in a location that **had 5 peak sun hours** per day of insolation and had **10% losses** from shading.

4kWac x 5PSH x 0.9 derating = 18kWh/day

PSH = Peak Sun Hours = Insolation is the amount of sunshine that you get in a particular location on the average day throughout the year at a particular tilt angle. PSH is usually between 4 and 6.

0.9 derating is from the 10% losses.

If you lose 10%, then you keep 90%.

Mathematically, 10%/100%=0.1 (turn percentage into a decimal)

Subtract that from 1.

1−0.1=0.9 derating factor.

Always think of what you are keeping with derating, not what you are losing.

Many people can look at a number, such as 89% and just write 0.89 without doing the math.

Practice test question:

A 7kWdc PV system makes 5.5kWac when 1000W per square meter are shining on it. If this is in a location that will get an average of 4.5 peak sun hours (PSH) per day and there are 12% losses from shading, then about how much energy will this system produce in a month?

a. 145GWh
b. 650kWh
c. 830kWh
d. 90kWh

> Derating for 12% means you keep 88%
>
> 1−0.12 = 0.88, which is decimal you keep 88%

Answer:

5.5kWac x 4.5PSH x 0.88 derating x 30 days

Explanation:

System makes 5.5kWac (inverter output) under "peak sun conditions" of 1000W per square meter.

There are 4.5 peak sun hours of insolation, which means that the solar radiation is equivalent to 4.5 hours of 1000 watts per square meter. This is like if it were **noon for 4.5 hours** and then dark the rest of the day.

12% losses means that we lose 12% and we keep 88% of our production. Losses + what we keep has to equal 100%. Percentages are decimals moved 2 places. 12%/100=0.12 and is the same as 12%. If we subtract 0.12 from 1 we get what we keep, which is 0.88 or 88%. One way to check our math here is adding 0.12 + 0.88 and we get 1.

We then multiply:

5.5kWac x 4.5PSH x 0.88 derating x 30 days = 653kWh

The answer in an exam can be rounded off to 650kWh.

SYSTEM LOSSES

There are always going to be losses and when you know how much solar energy lands on the PV array, then every step of the way, there are going to be losses. If you have a 10% efficient solar system powering a 10% efficient lightbulb, you would end up with 1% of the energy from the sunlight being turned back into light. This is an example that is not too far from reality with older technology.

Here is the math:

10% in decimal form is 0.1

0.1 x 0.1 = 0.01 = 1%

Using sunlight for lighting can be about 100 times more efficient than using PV and light bulbs.

There is a website put out by the US Government National Renewable Energy Labs (NREL) that is often used to size PV systems. At the older PVWATTS website we could see a table of various **derating factors**. Today they do it a little differently, but the old way is a good example for learning the math. Today the website shows you what you lose, rather than what you keep.

NREL PVWATTS websites: http://pvwatts.nrel.gov/

All of the derating factors can be multiplied together to come up with a single derating factor.

0.95 x 0.92 x 0.98 x 0.995 x 0.98 x 0.99 x 0.95 x 0.98 x 1.0 x 1.0 = 0.77

When all of the derating factors above are multiplied together, the system derate value will in this example be **0.77**, which means that the PV system will keep 77% of the energy or in other words lose 23% of the energy.

Unlike the previous example, these derating factors are from the dc STC wattage measurements of the PV modules to the ac kWh output. Every step along the way, you lose energy.

AC kWh output is what you want in the end and dc STC watts are how the PV modules are tested, rated and sold.

In the example above, the derating factor default value for shading is 1, which means that there is no shading. In most installations, there is some shade. Shading will sometimes be calculated with a shade measuring device, such as a Solmetric Suneye or a Solar Pathfinder. Often solar designers will use

Figure 7.1 PV system derating factors from National Renewable Energy Lab (NREL)

Component Derate Factors	Default Value	Allowed Range
PV module nameplate rating	0.95	0.800 - 1.050
Inverter and Transformer	0.92	0.88 - 0.98
Module mismatch	0.98	0.970 - 0.995
Diodes and connections	0.995	0.990 - 0.997
DC wiring losses	0.98	0.970 - 0.990
AC wiring losses	0.99	0.980 - 0.993
Array soiling	0.95	0.300 - 0.995
System availability	0.98	0.000 - 0.995
Array shading	1.000	0.000 - 1.000
Tracker misalignment	1.000	0.950 - 1.000

proprietary software to determine shading that uses data from laser assisted aerial surveys and satellites.

Other **parameters that effect production are tilt and azimuth, which are collectively called orientation**. Orientation's effect on production is most accurately calculated with software. There are however generalities or "rules of thumb" that are often used.

TILT

Latitude tilt is best for equinox time of the year (around March 21 or September 21). This is when the sun is directly over the equator. Also, latitude tilt is often good for annual production. 30-degree tilt is a good tilt for annual production for much of the latitudes of the United States, Europe, the Middle East and China.

Latitude +15 degrees tilt is best for winter and fall production. Often stand-alone PV systems are optimized for winter. If December were the month with worst inso-lation (solar energy), then we would call December the "**critical design month**".

Latitude −15 degrees tilt is best for summer and spring. This is when the sun is highest in the sky and decreasing the tilt is best.

A tilt that is close to zero can have trouble keeping clean, since the rain has trouble getting the dirt over the frame edge. Some designers do not tilt less than 5 or 10 degrees, so that PV modules will self-clean better in the rain. In locations without rain for a whole season, dirt can build up on the module, which we call **soiling**. If a PV module does not have a frame, it is called a **PV laminate** and will not be affected as much by flat or very low tilt angles, since the soiling will not build up on the glass by the module frames.

Often designers will design a system so that the tilt is less than optimal, so that they can fit more on the roof. **An increased tilt angle takes more room, due to inter-row shading**.

AZIMUTH (NORTH, SOUTH, EAST AND WEST)

In the northern hemisphere, we tend to get the most production with PV facing **south**. Often other than south orientations are acceptable, depending on the orientation of the roof and the price of the energy. If PV prices are low and energy prices are high, such as in Hawaii, there is a good argument for filling up every space on the roof.

PV prices falling opens up opportunities

As PV prices go down, we can re-evaluate the profitability of putting solar in places that we previously would not put solar. For example, I just put PV on my north roof. Five years ago, I would have never considered putting PV on my north facing roof, however PV prices have come down so much that the PV on my north roof was a better investment than the PV that I put on my south roof 5 years ago. The PV on the north roof is making two-thirds of what the PV on my south roof makes, but the PV on my south roof cost twice as much. If I put PV on my south, east or west walls, it would also make about two-thirds of what my south facing roof produces.

If people saw me put PV on my north facing roof 5 or 10 years ago, I would have been laughed at without being funny.

A reason to orient PV to the southwest is because of time-of-use (TOU) electricity rates. TOU rates make electricity more expensive in the afternoons when electricity demand is high and when the sun is moving to the west.

Here is a list of factors that would increase or decrease PV system output.

Increase output:

1. Cold temperatures (increases voltage)
   a. Increased airflow
   b. Space between PV and roof
   c. Cold climate
   d. High elevation

2. Clean PV (increases current)
   a. Rain recently
   b. Washing PV

3. Increased irradiance (increases current)
   a. Reflections
   b. High elevations

4. Efficient equipment
   a. Inverters
   b. Transformers
   c. Charge controllers

Decrease Output:

1. Soiling (decreases current)
   a. Dusty roads
   b. Farm animals

2. Snow on PV (decreases current)

3. Hot temperatures (decreases voltage)
   a. Lack of airflow
   b. BIPV (Building Integrated PV)

4. Voltage drop (wires too thin or long)
   a. Wire sizes: 2/0AWG > 1AWG > 10AWG

5. Loose wire connections

6. Shading

7. Inverter/equipment efficiency (inefficiency)

Practice question 1:

A 12kWdc PV system with 15% losses in a location with 4.8 Peak sun hours per day will make how much energy in a year?

12kWdc x 0.85 derating x 4.8 PSH x 365 = 17,870kWh per year

Practice question 2:

A PV system that makes 5kWac during peak sun conditions is in a location with 4.8 peak sun hours per day. How much energy will the system make in a month?

5kWac x 4.8PSH x 30 = 720kWh per month

Practice question 3:

A barn has a 100W light bulb that is on 100% of the time and a **746-watt (1 HP)** pump that is on 25% of the time. How much energy does it use in a week?

Light

100W x 24 hours x 7 days = 16,800Wh = 16.8kWh

> 746W = 1 Horsepower

Pump

746W x 24 hours x 0.25 x 7 days = 31,332Wh = 31.3 kWh

Light + Pump

16.8 kWh + 31.3kWh = 48.1kWh

Practice question 4:

If a 12V pump drew 5A for 2 hours, how much energy did it use and how many amp hours would it take from a 12V battery?

Energy calculation

12V x 5A x 2 hours = 120Wh (not kWh)

There are **different ways to calculate Ah** for this problem.

120Wh/12V = 10Ah
5A x 2 hours = 10Ah

Remember that Ah are just Amps x hours

Practice question 5:

Grid tied inverter size is based on?

a. Loads
b. PV array size in kW
c. PV array size in kWh
d. Charge controller

Explanation: A grid tied inverter will convert dc to ac at the rate of which the array is supplying power to the inverter. The inverter should be sized based on the array. In most instances, the inverter will be sized slightly smaller than the array. This is because the array is rated for dc STC watts and the inverter is rated for ac watts. **The grid tied inverter is sized based on the array size in kW.** Correct answer is b.

Practice question 6:

What would be the main benefit of oversizing a battery bank?

a. Increase in array kWh
b. Increase in days of autonomy
c. Decrease in array size
d. Decreased inverter size

Explanation: Increasing the size of the battery bank allows for more time with bad weather. Increasing your days of autonomy means that you can go more days without input from the sun. Autonomy means alone. **The main benefit of oversizing a battery bank is increasing days of autonomy.** Correct answer is b.

Practice question 7:

When sizing a **self-regulating PV system**, what criteria do you need to have in order to not need a charge controller?

a. Battery must be lithium ion
b. Battery bank must be less than array size
c. 1 hour charge is less than 3% of battery capacity
d. Battery must be Valve Regulated Lead Acid

Explanation: A self-regulating system does not have a charge controller and must not overcharge the battery. If a system is sized so that in **1 hour the battery will not get charged more than 3%** then this would be good for the battery. This is a rule spelled out in the National Electric Code. The correct answer is c.

Practice question 8:

Which 12kW system would produce the most energy?

a. BIPV
b. Flush mounted rooftop
c. Ground mount
d. Pole mount

Explanation: BIPV (Building Integrated PV) will have the least amount of air flow and operate the warmest and least efficient of the PV listed above. Then flush mounted rooftop, which is the typical residential solution, would be next on the list. Ground mount would produce even more and a **pole mount would operate best** of the above, because it would have the best airflow to release the heat away from the dark colored PV modules, so that they will be cooler and have more voltage. The correct answer is d.

Practice question 9:

How much 15% efficient PV will fit on 25 square meters of roof space?

a. 3.75MW
b. 4kW
c. 3750W
d. 55kW

Explanation: The average PV module installed is about 15% efficient. When we test PV, the input is 1000W/m². If the module is **15% efficient**, we would expect to get:

0.15 x 1000W/m² = 150W/ m²
150W/ m² x 25 m² = 3750W

The correct answer is c.

Practice question 10:

What is the simplest type of PV system?

a. Utility interactive
b. Stand-alone
c. Direct coupled
d. Multimodal

Explanation: Of the above answers, the most difficult is the multimodal. Multimodal means that it can work in utility interactive mode and stand-alone mode. Next on the list is stand-alone, since it is complicated to incorporate batteries. Utility interactive is next, since it has no battery or charger, but it does have an inverter. The simplest type of system is the direct-coupled system, which is just a load and a PV. It works when the sun is shining and does not when it is dark. A good example of this simple direct-coupled system is a solar attic fan.

PV system electrical design

SINGLE LINE DIAGRAMS

Single line diagrams (SLD), also known as one line diagrams, are diagrams showing how components are connected to each other. On the other hand, three line diagrams show more precisely how equipment are wired together. With every circuit, there are at least two and often three or more wires connecting the circuit and the grounding systems.

There are many different kinds of single and three line diagrams. Many three line diagrams have more than three lines. Some single line diagrams are very simple, such as the one shown in Figure 8.1, and others are more complex with a lot of equipment.

Figure 8.1 Single line diagram

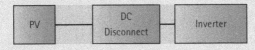

Figure 8.2 Three line diagram

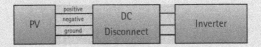

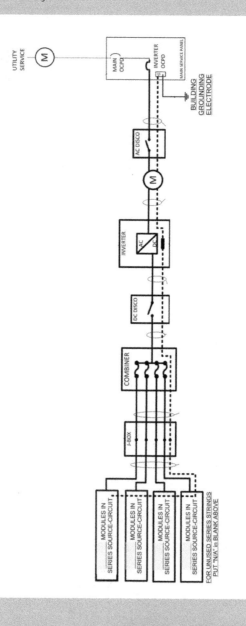

Figure 8.3 Single line diagram fill in forms adapted from www.solarabcs.org. The Solar America Board of Codes and Standards has an expedited permit process that is very helpful. Notice this drawing does not have separate lines for negative and positive.

To control undercharging of batteries, the power has to turn off when the voltage of the battery gets low. This **can be done by the inverter or the charge controller.**

Figure 8.4 Single line drawing of stand-alone setup

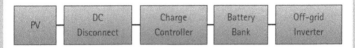

Whatever the **low voltage set point is will determine the wire size for the inverter input circuit (between the inverter and the battery).** An inverter will require more current at a lower inverter voltage set point since:

Voltage x Current = Power

Just remember, the lower the voltage, the higher the current and the bigger the wire required for an off-grid inverter input circuit.

Figure 8.5 Stand-alone inverter input circuit current determined by low voltage. Note: often charge controller is between battery and inverter.

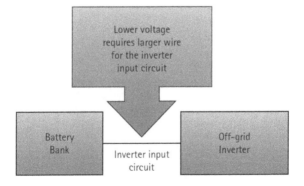

Figure 8.6 Series positive to negative increases voltage

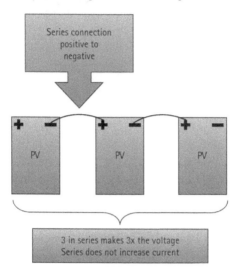

Figure 8.7 Parallel connections increase current not voltage

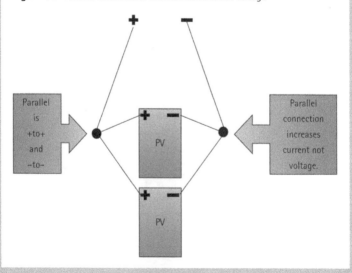

PV **source circuits** meet **PV output circuits** at the dc **combiner**. This is where the parallel PV dc circuit connections are made.

Ac combiner: There is no such thing as an ac combiner according to the National Electric Code; however when someone in the industry talks about an ac combiner, it is often a subpanel that is used for combining ac inverter circuits in parallel. Saying ac combiner is about as correct as saying solar panel when you mean solar module or saying string when you mean PV source circuit. It is done all the time and we know what they are talking about.

AMPACITY

The **ability** of a conductor (wire) to **carry current** is called **ampacity**.

When a conductor carries more current, it heats up. The insulation (like plastic) around the wire can only take so much heat. When a conductor carries too much current, it heats up beyond the temperature rating of the insulation of the conductor. The **temperature rating of the conductor affects ampacity**.

Factors that influence ampacity (ability of conductor to carry current):

1. Thickness of wire
2. Insulation around the wire
3. Hot temperatures
4. Airflow around wire.

OHM'S LAW AND VOLTAGE DROP

Ohm's Law states **V = IR**

V = Voltage
I = Current
R = Resistance

Voltage drop is when voltage and power are lost on a wire.

Voltage drop is reduced when the wire is either short or thick, which is why it is better to use thicker wires for better efficiency.

Because V = IR, if we have less current, then we will have less voltage drop. This means that **voltage and current are directly proportional** to each other according to Ohm's Law.

It should be obvious that having a short wire is good and having a thicker wire is more efficient.

Also, having higher voltage is more efficient, since Voltage × Current = Power and more voltage means less current for the same amount of power. This is why we have high voltage power lines.

Transformers change high voltage and low current to low voltage and high current. Transformers only work for alternating current (ac).

DC-to-dc converters (optimizers) can do the same thing as a transformer for direct current.

Most inverters used today are called functional grounded inverters. This means that there is a specific relationship between the voltage of ground, the equipment metal exposed parts and the current carrying conductors. Most inverters used today are the non-isolated types (formerly called ungrounded). These inverters usually work at voltages where the ground voltage is about in the middle of the positive and negative voltages. This is coordinated through the electronics of the inverter.

All inverters do have equipment grounding. Equipment grounding is a **green** wire or a **bare** copper wire and less often a **green wire with a yellow stripe**. Any exposed metal that may be subject to contact with a loose wire has to have equipment grounding to prevent shock.

> An dc disconnect connecting a PV circuit to an interactive inverter must open up both positive and negative and not just one or the other. This was not always the case and there are still very rare exceptions.

CHARGE CONTROLLERS

Charge controllers are only used with battery systems (something to charge).

Charge controllers are between the PV and the battery.

When a charge controller is used an inverter is usually not connected to the PV.

> Charge controllers are **not** used on **self-regulating PV systems** where the charging current in 1 hour is **less than 3%** of battery capacity.

AC AND DC COUPLED BATTERY SYSTEMS

Dc coupled systems are historically the typical battery based PV systems where PV is connected to a charge controller that charges a battery. The battery is often connected to a battery inverter through the charge controller that can power loads (devices that use energy) at night. A dc coupled system uses a charge controller that is connected to PV and an ac coupled system does not.

Ac coupled systems require two different kinds of inverters. They use PV connected interactive inverters (grid-tie style) that can be turned on by the "microgrid" created by another battery-based inverter. In a way, the battery-based inverter tricks the interactive inverter into thinking that there is a utility present in order to turn on the interactive inverter. Ac coupled systems can be made to convert an existing utility interactive system into a system that works on-and off-grid, which is also called a grid-tied battery backup system.

Ac and dc coupled systems can both be configured to work as grid-tied battery backup systems. Another name for this is a **multimodal** or **bimodal** system. This means it can work in utility interactive or stand-alone mode. When there is a utility outage, the multimodal inverter will power only loads that are isolated from the utility. A multimodal inverter will have at least two ac outputs, including one output that is interactive and will immediately disconnect from the grid when the grid goes down and another output that can power stand-alone loads in case of utility outage. The stand-alone output can also work when the grid-tied output is functioning.

BATTERY CHARGING STAGES

Bulk is charging fast and done first.

Absorption charge is slowing down the charge.

Float charge is a trickle charge to keep the battery charged.

Equalization charging is for battery maintenance and is the **highest voltage** charge.

Equalization charges are only done to flooded lead-acid batteries which are NOT sealed and that are NOT maintenance-free. Maintenance-free batteries are not equalized, since we cannot add distilled water to sealed batteries to replace the water that was split into hydrogen and oxygen during the equalization process. When batteries are overcharged, H_2O is split into hydrogen and oxygen gasses via a process called electrolysis.

TYPICAL USA UTILITY PARAMETERS

Frequency 60 cycles per second (hertz or Hz)

Residential 120/240V split phase/single phase

Commercial 3-phase voltages:

    120/208V
    277/480V
    240V
    480V

If you ask an honest electrician how long it takes to learn about 3-phase power, they will tell you they are still learning, so do not get discouraged. Only Nikola Tesla truly understood.

Just like an inverter input has a voltage range, so do your electronics. Most computer and phone chargers will work at all plug outlets voltages around the world. Somewhere on the charger it will tell you the voltage range. This computer works from 100 to 250V at 50- and 60-hertz.

In most of the world, including most of Asia, Africa, Middle East and Europe, the frequency of the grid is 50-hertz and there are no North American split phase voltages. Entering a house in most of the world is about 220V to 240V to every outlet and appliance. 230V multiplied by the square root of 3 is about 400V, so it is often called 230/400V 3-phase going into large buildings or 240/415V 3-phase.

The Philippines has a mixture of both worlds, since it used to be part of the United States, there is a 60-hertz frequency and voltages less similar to the US.

Canada is mostly like the US, but with 346/600V 3-phase.

Latin America is more like the US until you get further into South America.

OVERCURRENT PROTECTION DEVICES (OCPD)

Two types of OCPD are fuses and circuit breakers.

OCPDs protect conductors and equipment from overcurrents by opening the circuit when the current is too much. (Opening a circuit is how things are turned off.)

Maximum Series Fuse Rating is what is specified on the back of a PV module along with rated power, open circuit voltage (Voc), maximum power voltage (Vmp), short circuit current (Isc) and maximum power current (Imp). The maximum series fuse rating means that if you had a fuse with a higher current rating, it would not protect the PV module. In a way, the maximum series fuse rating is like the "ampacity" of the PV module. Often PV modules have a maximum series fuse rating of 15A or 20A.

Module interconnects connect the modules together and can be made with **USE-2** wire or **PV wire**.

VOLTAGE RANGES

Equipment that PV is connected to and that process power, such as **inverters and charge controllers**, will have a voltage range for operation. If the voltage is too low, then the equipment will not turn on. If the voltage is too high, then it can damage the equipment or be dangerous.

The voltage ranges are specified for the equipment on labels and datasheets.

VOLTAGE AND TEMPERATURE CALCULATIONS

The most difficult concept to master in this book is what is commonly called "string sizing". What we will do is figure out what the voltage will be when the voltage goes up when it is cold or what the voltage will be when it is hot.

When it is **hot and the voltage gets low**, we run the risk of the system not turning on or producing ineffectively, which is not a safety problem, but a waste.

When it gets too **cold, the voltage will get higher** and it is possible that on a cold day the PV system will have enough voltage to destroy equipment, void the warranty of the inverter, cause a fire or violate the codes and standards. Overvoltage is a safety issue.

There are different ways of determining how voltage changes with respect to temperature. The main way that this is done is with what is called a temperature coefficient for voltage.

Coefficients are also used for other things in science and with the electricity.

EXAMPLES OF COEFFICIENTS

Expansion of metal: Metal expands a certain amount for each degree warmer it gets. We can use the coefficients for the expansion of aluminum and steel when designing our PV racks, rails and conduit.

Atmospheric pressure: For every meter rise in elevation, you have less atmosphere. This can be important when designing a high-altitude PV system.

We can even have coefficients for making coffee. For every six cups of water, we use one scoop of ground coffee. If we want 24 cups of coffee, then we need three scoops. We could say the coefficient is one sixth of a scoop per cup of coffee or 0.167 scoops per cup (forgive me if you like it stronger).

PV and voltage

Now let's think of PV and voltage. In general PV open circuit **voltage (Voc) goes up about one third of a percent for every 1°C** decrease in temperature.

Since all of the PV is tested at Standard Test Conditions (**STC**) **at 25°C** then at 24°C we would gain one third of a percent of our voltage. One third of a percent is represented as 0.33%/°C. If our voltage was 100V then one third of a percent of 100V is one third of 1, since one percent of 100 is 1.

One third of 1 is 0.33, so at 24° our 100V would go up to 100.33V.

If our temperature went down ten times that much or ten degrees less than 25°C to 15°C, then ten times a third is ten thirds or 10 × 0.33 = 3.3% increase in Voc.

3.3% of 100V is 3.3V, so then our new voltage at 15°C would be 103.3Voc.

If we really thought about it and our temperature coefficient for voltage is a third of a percent for each 1°C, then for every 3°C is a 1% change.

What we are going to do now is a practice problem. This will seem difficult the first time so do not get discouraged. Once you get the system down, you may think it is easy.

Given:

PV Voc = 40V
Temp Coefficient for Voc = −0.3%/°C
Cold Temperature = −5°C

What will be the voltage of the module at −5C?

Change in temperature from 25°C to −5°C is 30°C less than 25°C STC.

(+5C would only be 20°C less than 25°C STC)

Multiply change in temperature by temperature coefficient:

30°C x 0.3%/°C = 9% increase in voltage

Using common sense

Most books teach people to calculate the Voc by subtracting the STC of 25°C from the cold temperature, which often means that you are subtracting a positive number from a negative number to get a more negative number and then multiplying that resulting negative number by a negative number which is the temperature coefficient of Voc. I prefer to use common sense, so we do not get lost in a formula. Common sense indicates that if it gets colder than 25°C, then our voltage is going up. Common sense also tells us that if our cold temperature is below zero, then our change in temperature will be greater than 25°C and we can just add the numbers together ignoring negative and positive, so we added 5 + 25 in our example to get 30°C. If our cold temperature was greater than 0°C, then we can just subtract our cold temperature from 25°C. STC is always 25°C, so we have to memorize 25°C.

Use common sense every step of the way and mentally check your steps to make sure they make sense. We all make mistakes and common sense will tell us to go back and repeat a step if it is way off.

A 9% increase in voltage can be found by multiplying the voltage by 0.09.

We get 0.09 by moving the decimal 2 places to the left or by dividing 9% by 100.

0.09 x 40V = 3.6V increase in Voc (when cold)

We can then add 3.6V to 40V to get our voltage

40Voc + 3.6V = 43.6Voc (cold)

A short cut to doing this is to multiply our voltage by 1.09 instead of 0.09 to get our final voltage.

40Voc x 1.09 = 43.6Voc cold temperature

43.6V is our open circuit voltage (Voc) at our cold temperature of –5°C.

The next question: What is the maximum number of PV modules can we put in series? We first need to know the maximum acceptable voltage at the input of the inverter (or charge controller).

Inverter maximum input voltage is 1000V

To determine how many modules can be in series without exceeding 1000V

1000V/43.6V = 22.9 modules

Since we cannot cut a module in half or go over voltage, then we will **always round down when determining maximum number of modules in series**.

> If you are using high temperatures and determining minimum number of modules in series, you will round up.

The maximum number of modules in series in this example is 22 in series. 23 in series would bring the voltage up over 1000V on a cold day and void the warranty of the inverter or worse.

> Engineering supervision
>
> Under engineering supervision, it is possible to use another method using advanced calculations that could possibly let someone have more modules in series due to solar irradiance raising the solar cell temperature. To learn this method, I highly encourage you to believe in yourself and become an engineer.

At the end of this book, there will be a special section on doing voltage temperature calculations where we will study this concept more and learn more shortcuts!

Chapter 9

PV system mechanical design

PV mounting systems affect performance due to:

1. Airflow
   a. More airflow is better and will cause heat to leave PV and make voltage higher. High voltage means more power and energy because:
      i. **Volts × Amps = Power**
      ii. **Power × Time = Energy**

2. Orientation
   a. Residential roof mounts usually go with the slope of the roof. **When a system goes with the slope of the roof, we call that flush mounted.** In most parts of the USA a **30-degree sloped PV system facing south is close to optimal.** Often times latitude tilt is also close to optimal. As the price of PV decreases we see every slope of a roof having flush mounted PV going with the slope of the roof.
   b. Repeating rows take inter-row shading into consideration. When the tilt is less, more PV will fit because of less inter-row shading with decreased tilt and module height.
   c. Flat or very low-sloped PV systems will have trouble staying clean and will have soiling or will have trouble shedding snow. PV laminates are modules without frames and are often the preferred choice for flat mounted PV systems, since having frames will cause dirty water puddles on flat installed modules. Most PV modules have aluminium frames.

Building Integrated PV (BIPV) is PV that is part of the roofing or building materials. BIPV typically does not have airflow, so will operate at a higher temperature, which will slightly decrease performance when compared to systems that have airflow. BIPV is more expensive and less common than mass-produced PV modules.

Figure 9.1 BIPV
Source: ©2014 Tony Diaz, Century Roof and Solar

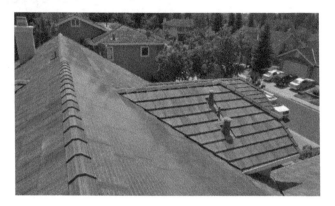

Flush Mounted PV usually has three inches to six inches between the PV and the roof. The six inches keeps the PV cooler than BIPV and will also keep the roof and the attic cooler than if the sunlight was hitting the roof directly. Flush mounted PV is the predominant residential sloped roof PV mounting system.

Flush mounted PV mounting systems:

1. Composition asphalt shingle mounting
2. Tile mounting
3. Metal roof mounting
4. Wood shake shingles.

Waterproofing is always a concern when putting holes into a roof and there are many different types of systems used to waterproof roof penetrations.

Flashing is strongly recommended. Flashing is overlapping materials to prevent water intrusion.

Low slope roof mounting is the typical **commercial roof** mounting system. A low slope roof is often called a flat roof, although it is never completely flat so that rainwater will drain from the roof.

There are two predominant types of low slope roof mounting systems:

1. **Ballasted systems** are **not structurally attached** to the roof with penetrations (holes). Ballasted systems are designed so that something heavy is put onto the PV system to hold it down. Often concrete rectangular blocks called paving stones are used. Ballasted systems are often not used when the roof cannot take the extra weight or where there is a lot of wind. However, there have been ballasted systems that successfully made it through hurricanes. Ballasted racking systems are often designed in wind tunnels and often include wind deflectors to keep them stable.

2. **Penetrating systems** use structural attachments, usually called posts, jacks, standoffs or pedestals, that attach the racking system to a strong part of the roof. A strong part of the roof is usually a purlin, a truss or a rafter, which can take the forces of the PV system. It is not good to attach the PV system to something not as strong, such as the roof deck. Most residential systems are also penetrating systems and attach to the roof via structural attachments.

Figure 9.2 Flush mounted composition asphalt shingle PV mounting system with flashing. Flashing is overlapping of materials to prevent water intrusion. Figure shows QuickMountPV flashing with IronRidge rail system.
Source: Courtesy Quick Mount PV

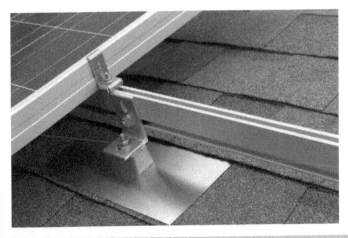

Figure 9.3 Ballasted system
Source: Courtesy Advanced Solar Products, Solstice Mounting System.

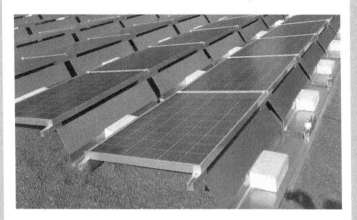

3. **Combination ballast and penetrations**. Often engineers will put as much weight as the roof can handle and then put some penetrations around the corners where the most wind uplift forces are. (Wind uplift forces in North America are measured in pounds per square foot.)

Ground mount PV systems contain most of the PV installed in the world today in large "Utility Scale" solar farms. Ground mounts take up valuable real estate and are not as common in cities. Ground mounts come in all sizes from less than a kW to thousands of MWs. A thousand megawatts is one gigawatt.

Ground mounted systems can be mass-produced with increased efficiencies.

Ground mounts have increased airflow beyond roof mounted systems, which means slightly greater voltage, power and energy.

Pole mounted PV systems are PV arrays that are put up on a single pole. They have **more airflow than ground mount, and roof mounted systems** but are more difficult to engineer. Pole mounted systems can more easily fall over if not secured properly.

Tracking systems follow the path of the sun for increased production. As the price of PV goes down, the need for tracking systems decreases. When PV was expensive every extra kWh of energy that we could get out of a module was important. Now that PV is less expensive, it is often a better value proposition to buy more PV than to buy a tracker. Trackers are also known for being high maintenance.

All of that being said, the most popular tracker used today is a **single-axis tracker** that will face east in the morning, west in the evening and will be flat at noon. This is called a **horizontal axis tracker** and often used with large utility scale PV systems.

A **2-axis tracker** will be mounted on a pole mount and **follow the sun in every direction exactly**. 2-axis trackers are not common these days, since they require maintenance and it can be less expensive to buy more PV than to pay for maintenance. 2-axis trackers were more popular in the past when PV was more expensive.

Concentrating PV is PV that uses magnifying lenses or mirrors to focus light onto an efficient solar cell. Concentrating PV **usually has a 2-axis tracker** to accurately track the sun in order for the concentrating PV to work well.

Sealants are used to keep the roof waterproof. The most popular sealants used are **polyurethane and silicone**. Polyurethane is the most common sealant, since it is the best sealant.

All sealants can degrade in sunlight, which is why roofing best practices do not depend upon sealants for the only source of leak protection.

Fasteners are used to fasten the mechanical racking systems. **Stainless steel fasteners** are usually used and most importantly used in **humid, moist or marine environments** where corrosion is more likely.

Different forces are considered when mounting PV systems. Some of these forces are wind loads, snow loads, seismic loads, live loads and dead loads.

Wind loads are measured in **pounds per square foot (Psf)** in the USA. Wind loads are worse in different parts of the roof. Typically, the corners are worse, the edges are next and the middle of the roof is the safest place for PV. Also, urban areas are safer than wide open areas due to wind. Increased module tilt causes more forces on the PV from the wind.

Snow loads add extra weight. Roofs in these areas are often not able to take extra weight from ballasted PV systems. **Structural engineers** often have to qualify a roof for a PV system in areas with high snow loads. Lower tilt

Figure 9.4 Piles
Source: Photo by Sean White, 2010 Sarnia Solar Project

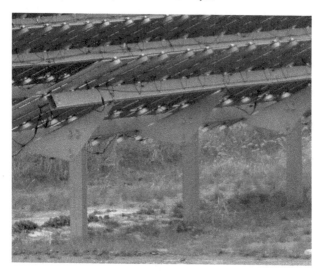

angles are often used in areas with snow loads, since high tilt angles can cause build-up of snow on the roof, which can be too much weight for the roof.

Dead loads are loads that are **permanent** on the roof, such as the solar system you install and anything that is part of the building.

Live loads are **temporary** and include workers on the roof and snow falling on the roof.

Piles are used in most utility scale PV systems. Piles are typically pieces of steel that are driven into the earth with a pile driver that is specially made for PV projects.

Smaller ground-mounts usually do not use piles, since the cost of bringing a pile driver to a small job would be cost prohibitive and then concrete is used in the ground according to racking manufacturer's instructions.

Ground screws, also known as **earth screws** are also used in some large solar projects. Think of a 6 foot (2 meter) long screw that is screwed into the earth. Piles are better at breaking through rocks in the earth than ground screws.

Chapter 10

Performance analysis, maintenance and troubleshooting

If we have a good grasp of the previous nine chapters, this chapter will be common sense.

Many PV systems were installed incorrectly and many others were installed in ways that will not last the test of time. Due to the rapid growth of PV installations, most of the equipment installed in the world is less than three years old. As equipment ages, it will have problems that need fixing.

Commissioning a PV system is what is done after the system is installed. There are different levels of commissioning. Just turning the system on after checking voltage is the simplest form of commissioning, but usually when someone talks about commissioning a system, especially a large system, they measure irradiance data in the **plane of the array (tilt and azimuth orientation)** with an irradiance-measuring device called a **pyranometer**. Also, they measure the solar cell temperature. Then calculations are done to correct for temperature and irradiance, in order to see that the PV system is working as it should. A common mistake people make is assuming that a 7kW PV system with a 6kW inverter should be making 6 or 7kWac when the system is powered up. More often a PV system will be making half of its rated power rather than its full rated power. This is because clouds, time of day and various derating factors, including solar cell temperature, irradiance, soiling, inverter inefficiency and voltage drop, will reduce the amount of energy produced. I have never seen a PV system make as much power as the PV was rated for. Perhaps in a very cold bright place, such as the top of Mt. Everest it could be possible.

Another common reason that a PV system is not turning on is because the system needs to be turned on for five minutes before it will export power to the grid. This is because of the anti-islanding requirements of utility interactive inverters. All interactive inverters must sample the grid before connecting. We do not want an inverter to feed a dirty grid.

Monitoring is very common with PV systems. Often residential monitoring consists of a device that measures current and voltage on the ac output of the inverter and relays that information via the Internet.

Monitoring for larger systems often has more parameters that are measured, such as wind speed, solar cell temperature and irradiance. Some monitoring is on the PV source circuit (string) level and other monitoring would be on the inverter output level.

When diagnosing a problem on a PV system, make sure to **stay safe**. This means looking at your system first, turning things off with disconnects and then taking measurements and saving the corrections for last when you know what is wrong. Always remember to be safe! Making sure that your voltmeter works before testing with it is standard practice.

Common performance issues:

1. PV system turns off on hot sunny days.
    a. Problem is voltage gets too low when temperature gets too hot.
    b. Correction is putting more modules in series to raise voltage or getting another inverter with a lower voltage input window.
2. Ground fault detected.
    a. Likely a fault on a source circuit (string).
    b. Measure voltages on separate PV source circuits to find ground fault.
    c. Make sure everything has been turned off first.
    d. Be careful of getting shocked.
3. Blown fuse in a combiner.
    a. Likely positive to negative short circuit.
    b. Multiple strings feeding backwards through one fuse in a combiner.
    c. Carefully correct the problem after visually determining what is wrong and turning everything off.
    d. Find the fault and correct the problem being careful to not get shocked.

When no fuses are required

Most string inverters do not use fuses, since when there are 1 or 2 PV source circuits going to a single MPPT, then fusing is not required. If there were a short circuit with 1 or 2 PV source circuits, there would not be enough current to blow the fuse, so having a fuse would be misleading and a false sense of security, besides costing extra.

4. Performance is not good for a few days in the winter according to monitoring.
    a. Look for snow or bad weather.
    b. Solution is to wait or move snow.
5. In a dry climate performance is worse at the middle or end of the dry season.
    a. Look for soiling (dirt).
    b. Solution is to wash modules.
    c. Check for low operating voltage problems due to heat on array.
    d. Check for excessive voltage due to undersized conductors.

Battery maintenance:

1. Check voltage with volt meter.
2. Clean terminals and equipment.
3. Check connections.
4. Inspect fuses and disconnects.
5. Inspect ventilation system.
6. Perform load test.

Battery maintenance for flooded lead acid batteries that are NOT sealed (NOT maintenance free):

1. Check fluid levels.
2. Replace missing fluid with distilled water.
3. Check specific gravity of battery acid.
    a. Hydrometer checks battery acid with a density test
    b. Refractometer checks battery acid with a test to see how light bends in fluid.
4. **Equalization charge** is a controlled overcharge for maintenance of non-sealed flooded lead acid batteries. Equalization charge splits H_2O and releases bubbles of hydrogen and oxygen, which will stir up the battery.

TEST TAKING STRATEGY

When taking a NABCEP exam, every question has four possible answers: a, b, c or d.

- Use common sense. Many times you can rule out most answers without even doing the calculation. The wrong answers will have the wrong units, be in the opposite direction or obviously be way off.
- No more than one answer can be correct, so if there are two answers that mean the same thing, then probably they are both wrong.
- There will be no "all of the above" choices.
- Write notes so you can go back at the end and see if you have a different perspective. Many questions have answers to other problems in them.
- Remember that complex math is a series of simple problems.
- Math can be done in different ways.
- You should have plenty of time, so be patient and do not let a tough question destroy your confidence. You do not have to get everything correct to pass.
- For math problems, practice with real equations: do not expect to read a book and then be able to work equations without practicing.
- Take the exam well rested and if you consume caffeine on a regular basis, try not to have too much or too little.
- State dependent memory: study at the same time of day and conditions that you take your exam.
- If you cannot do voltage temperature correction math, you can still pass the exam.
- Have confidence!

String sizing

**Knowing how many modules
to put in series using voltage
temperature calculations**

The most difficult part about this book will be learning to do the voltage temperature correction math. If you are overwhelmed with math, you can review this chapter and come back to it later. It is best to practice working sample questions in order to learn these concepts. Remember, these problems are a few simple calculations done in a pattern. The more you practice, the more confidence you will have.

For crystalline PV, Voc goes up about a third of a percent for every decrease of 1°C in temperature under 25°C.

A change of 1°C is a change of 1.8°F °Cs are bigger than °Fs

That means if it gets to be 3°C colder than 25°C then the change in temperature is going to be −3°C when it is 22°C.

A −3°C change with a third of a percent change in voltage for each degree C would mean:

3°C x one third percent per degree = 1% change

Since it is getting colder, that percentage will be a 1% increase in voltage.

6 degrees colder is a 2% increase in Voc

9 degrees colder is a 3% increase in Voc

12 degrees colder is a 4% increase in Voc

24 degrees colder than 25°C is 1°C

24 degrees colder is an 8% increase in Voc

These changes above are for a one-third percent coefficient. Sometimes the coefficients are different, but at least these examples are in the same ballpark. On an exam, if you are in the right ballpark, you have a good chance of answering a multiple-choice question correctly. In the field or on your desk at work, knowing the right range of answers is very helpful.

Here is another way of thinking of coefficients:

Say that all you had were t-shirts and for each 3 degrees below 25°C you had to put on another T-shirt to keep warm. How many shirts would you have to put on to keep warm at −5°C?

Answer:

- −5°C is 30 degrees colder than 25°C
- 30°C/3°C per shirt = 10 shirts

When we design our systems, we have to determine how many modules we can connect in series, so as to not go over voltage. Going over voltage can break whatever your PV is connected to. Inverters, charge controllers, wires, disconnects and all electrical equipment have voltage limits, which we cannot exceed safely.

If we put too many PV modules in series, then on a cold day when voltage is higher, it can ruin an inverter. We always have to design our systems so that we do not have too many PV modules in series. We call this string sizing.

The information that we use for string sizing is:

1. **Cold expected temperature**
2. **Temperature coefficient Voc**
3. **Voc of PV module**
4. **Maximum input voltage of inverter (or charge controller)**

Coldest expected temperature **many people get from www.solarabcs.org**.

Temperature coefficient of Voc is read from the datasheet/cutsheet. This is usually close to a third of a percent per degree C or −0.33%/°C.

Voc of PV module is found on the back of the module, the datasheet or many other places.

Maximum inverter input voltage is found on inverter documentation, cut-sheet or label on the inverter.

Here is how to do the math!

Steps:

1. **Find Delta T** (delta means difference)
   a. Determine difference in temperature from 25°C

2. **Multiply Delta T x Temp coefficient Voc**
   a. You then get % increase in voltage

3. **Determine increase in voltage**
   a. Think of this like sales tax
      i. 10% increase multiple by 1.1
      ii. 8% increase multiple by 1.08

4. **Max input voltage/cold temp PV voltage**
   a. Determines number of modules in series
   b. Divide cold temperature
   c. Always round down for cold temperatures, since rounding up would give you too much voltage.

Sample problem:

Given:

1. Cold temperature   −15°C
2. Temperature Coef Voc   −0.33%/°C
3. Voc   35Voc
4. Inverter Max input voltage 600V

How many is the most modules that can be configured in series?

15°C + 25°C = 40°C (Delta T)

> To make math more understandable and to find difference from 25°C, you can add numbers less than zero to 25 and subtract numbers greater than zero from 25.

0.132 + 1 = 1.132 (multiplying by 1.132 gives us a 13.2% increase)
1.132 × 35Voc = 39.62Voc cold
600V/39.62V = 15.14
15 in series max

> 40°C × 0.003/°C = 0.132 increase Voc
>
> We are turning percentages into decimals here by moving the decimal 2 places to the left in order to more easily do the math. We are also ignoring the fact that the coefficient is a negative number and just using the common sense that the voltage goes up when it becomes colder than 25°C.

Let's break this down simple style and get the hang of it quick:

Example:
Cold Temperature = −5°C
Temp Coef. Voc = −0.3%/°C
Voc = 40V
Inverter max input = 500V

Solar PV Basics patented string sizing shortcut

This way you do not need to use paper to write anything down.

Enter in your calculator:
5 + 25 = 30°C
30 × .003 = 0.09
0.09 + 1 = 1.09
1.09 × 40V = 43.6V
43.6V/500V = 0.0872
0.0872 then press 1/X button = 11.5

11 in series maximum

Division shortcut

You can see that part of the shortcut included doing division upside down when we divided 43.6V/500V rather than 500V/43.6V. This gives us the inverse (upside down fraction) of the answer we wanted, so all we have to do is to press the 1/X button on our calculator to flip the fraction back over. If you are using your phone for a calculator, try turning your phone sideways to get the extra functions on your calculator. If you do not have a 1/X button, then just do the division the normal way and divide 500V/43.6V in this example.

The best way to learn this is by repeating it many times right now. Here are some data and answers are on page 132. Solve for max modules in series.

Question 1:
1. Cold temperature   −10°C
2. Temperature Coef Voc   −0.33%/°C
3. Voc   35Voc
4. Inverter Max input voltage 600V

Question 2:
1. Cold temperature   +10°C
2. Temperature Coef Voc   −0.34%/°C
3. Voc   40Voc
4. Inverter Max input voltage 750V

Question 3:
1. Cold temperature   −20°C
2. Temperature Coef Voc   −0.3%/°C
3. Voc   37Voc
4. Inverter Max input voltage 1000V

Question 4:
1. Cold temperature   −7°C
2. Temperature Coef Voc   −0.31%/°C
3. Voc   44Voc
4. Inverter Max input voltage 1500V

Question 5:
1. Cold temperature   5°C
2. Temperature Coef Voc   −0.35%/°C
3. Voc   22Voc
4. Inverter Max input voltage 550V

Question 6:
1. Cold temperature   −40°C
2. Temperature Coef Voc   −0.29%/°C
3. Voc   36Voc
4. Inverter Max input voltage 1000V

Answers:

Question 1:
1. Cold temperature   −10°C
2. Temperature Coef Voc   −0.33%/°C
3. Voc   35Voc
4. Inverter Max input voltage 600V

$10 + 25 = 35C$
$35 \times .0033 = 0.1155$
$0.1155 + 1 = 1.1155$
$1.1155 \times 35V = 39V$
$39V/600V = 0.0651$
0.0651 press $1/X = 15.4$

Answer: 15 in series maximum

Question 2:

1. Cold temperature   +10°C
2. Temperature Coef Voc   −0.34%/°C
3. Voc   40Voc
4. Inverter Max input voltage   750V

$25 - 10 = 15°C$

$15 \times .0034 = 0.051$

$0.051 + 1 = 1.051$

$1.051 \times 40V = 42.04V$

$42.04V / 750V = 0.05605$

0.05605 press $1/X = 17.8$

Answer: 17 in series maximum

Question 3:

1. Cold temperature   −20°C
2. Temperature Coef Voc   −0.3%/°C
3. Voc   37Voc
4. Inverter Max input voltage   1000V

$20 + 25 = 45°C$

$45 \times .003 = 0.135$

$0.135 + 1 = 1.135$

$1.135 \times 37V = 41.995V$

$41.995V / 1000V = 0.041995$

0.041995 press $1/X = 23.8$

Answer: 23 in series maximum

Question 4:

1. Cold temperature   −7°C
2. Temperature Coef Voc   −0.31%/°C
3. Voc   44Voc
4. Inverter Max input voltage   1500V

7 + 25 = 32°C
32°C x .0031 = 0.0992
0.0992 + 1 = 1.0992
1.0992 x 44V = 48.3648V
48.3648V/1500V = 0.0322
0.0322 press 1/X = 31.06

Answer: 31 in series maximum

Question 5:

1. Cold temperature   5°C
2. Temperature Coef Voc   −0.35%/°C
3. Voc   22Voc
4. Inverter Max input voltage   550V

25 − 5 = 20°C
20°C x .0035 = 0.07
0.07 + 1 = 1.07
1.07 x 22V = 23.54V
23.54V/550V = 0.0428
0.0428 press 1/X = 23.4

Answer: 23 in series maximum

Question 6:
1. Cold temperature   −40°C
2. Temperature Coef Voc   −0.29%/°C
3. Voc   36Voc
4. Inverter Max input voltage   1000V

$40 + 25 = 65°C$
$65°C \times .0029 = 0.1885$
$0.1885 + 1 = 1.1885$
$1.1885 \times 36V = 42.786V$
$42.786V/1000V = 0.042786$
0.042786 press $1/X = 23.4$

Answer: 23 in series maximum

String sizing can also be done for hot temperatures. String sizing for hot temperatures determines the shortest string. If a string is too short, the inverter will not have enough voltage. This is not a safety issue, just not a good idea to have your inverter not turn on. Since it is not a safety issue, it is not a Code issue. When doing the math for a hot temperature you would use the Vmp, because that is the low voltage and we use a temperature coefficient for Vmp for hot temperatures. Also, we are going to find the shortest string and round up rather than down to have enough voltage. Additionally, the PV often operates 20°C to 30°C hotter than ambient because it is sitting in the sun.

Example of calculation for hot temperature correction for low voltage:
1. Hot PV cell temperature   60°C
2. Temperature Coef Vmp   −0.4%/°C
3. Vmp   30Vmp
4. Inverter Min input voltage   250V

$60°C − 25°C = 35°C$ (Delta T)
$35°C \times .004 = 0.14$ means 14% decrease in Vmp
$1 − 0.14 = 0.86$ is derating factor (for 14% decrease)
$0.86 \times 30Vmp = 25.8Vmp$ hot
$250V/25.8V = 9.7$

10 in series minimum to keep voltage high enough on a hot day

Seventy practice exam questions

Chapter 12

The NABCEP Entry Level Exam is a timed test, which you will be given 2 hours to complete.

There are two exams that are intended to prepare you for the NABCEP Associate exam. The first exam, in this chapter, is 70 questions, just like the NABCEP Associate exam. Detailed explanations and answers follow the 70 questions. The second exam can be found on the companion website for this book: www. routledge.com/Solar-Photovoltaic-Basics-A-Study-Guide-for-the-NABCEP-Associate-Exam/White/p/book/9781138102866. This is a more difficult exam, which covers good practice and knowledge gathering, and will hopefully make the NABCEP Associate exam seem easy. It can also be found on the following website: www.heatspring.com/sean

You may commence now!

1. An off-grid installation has a 1HP pump that is on 10% of the time and a 20W light that is on 100% of the time. What is the energy use per month?
   a. 54Wh
   b. 68kW
   c. 68kWh
   d. 0.63 MWh

2. What kind of ground faults do most inverters detect?
   a. High voltage
   b. Medium voltage
   c. Ac
   d. Dc

3. Current carrying ability of a conductor (wire) is called
  a. Ampacity
  b. Amps
  c. Inductance
  d. Insolation

4. According to Ohm's Law and voltage drop, the relationship between voltage drop and current is
  a. Proportional
  b. Inversely proportional
  c. Directly inverse
  d. Inversely direct

5. An Array in Sacramento California in August (hot and dry) is not producing as expected. Which of the following is NOT a likely problem?
  a. Decreased ac wire size and voltage loss
  b. String size too short
  c. String size too long
  d. Soiling

6. When using a digital multimeter, what is the first thing you should do?
  a. Turn the meter on
  b. Inspect the meter
  c. Touch the black lead to the white wire
  d. Touch the black lead to the black wire

7. Which is the worst design error?
  a. BIPV on a commercial job
  b. A fast growing tree to the north of the array in Idaho
  c. PV at 5-degree tilt at 40 degrees latitude
  d. Different tilt angles in a PV source circuit

8. The low design temperature is $-20°C$ and the Voc temperature correction factor for your PV is $-0.34\%/°C$. The characteristics of your module are Isc = 8A, Voc = 37V and Vmp = 29V. How many modules can you put in series for an inverter that cannot go over 500V?

    a. 10
    b. 11
    c. 12
    d. 13

9. MPPT is for

    a. Optimizing energy from the utility
    b. Getting the most energy from a battery with a MPPT inverter
    c. Optimizing power from a PV array
    d. Tracking the sun with a 2-axis tracker

10. Concentrated PV

    a. Only works with direct sunlight
    b. Usually has a single axis tracker
    c. Will get 30% power during cloudy conditions
    d. Is using heat to make electricity

11. Fall protection should be used at heights over

    a. 4 feet
    b. 2 feet
    c. 3 feet
    d. 6 feet

12. Parallel PV circuit connections increase

    a. Voltage
    b. Current
    c. Resistance
    d. EMF

13. Optimal tilt for off-grid PV system in the winter

    a. Latitude
    b. Latitude -15 degrees
    c. Latitude $+15$ degrees
    d. Vertical

14. What is the most acceptable rating of an enclosure for exposed circuit conductors mounted on an outside wall?
   a. NEMA 3R
   b. NEMA 11
   c. NEMA 4X
   d. NEMA 12

15. Bypass diodes are located in the
   a. Combiner box
   b. Inverter
   c. Wiring harness
   d. PV module

16. A PV array at a higher elevation would tend to produce more
   a. Current
   b. Heat
   c. Resistance
   d. Polysilicon

17. Voc = 36V, low temp = −2°C, inverter maximum input voltage = 500V temp coefficient of voltage = −0.35%/°C. What is the maximum number of modules that can be connected in series?
   a. 13
   b. 10
   c. 11
   d. 12

18. How much 14% efficient PV fits on 25 square meters?
   a. 3000W
   b. 4.5kW
   c. 4000W
   d. 3.5kW

19. Which is the smallest conductor?
   a. 18 AWG
   b. 10 AWG
   c. 0 AWG
   d. 3/0 AWG

20. Which of the following is the simplest type of PV system?
   a. Utility interactive
   b. Stand-alone
   c. Self-regulating
   d. Direct coupled

21. Sun path charts differ based on
   a. Longitude
   b. Latitude
   c. Azimuth
   d. Tilt angle

22. Series connections increase
   a. Voltage
   b. Current
   c. Cold
   d. Heat

23. The longest shadow at 2PM would be on
   a. June 1
   b. November 12
   c. February 14
   d. March 29

24. What is the ground mount advantage over a rooftop system?
   a. Takes no extra real estate
   b. Cooler
   c. Increased photosynthesis
   d. Soiling

25. Which test conditions have higher voltage?
   a. STC
   b. PTC
   c. CEC
   d. NOCT

26. Which is the best tilt angle for annual production in most of the USA (temperate latitudes)?

   a. Latitude +15 degrees

   b. Latitude – 15 degrees

   c. 30 degrees

   d. Longitude tilt

27. A 100kW STC PV system with 8% system losses, using PV that is +3 – 0% production tolerance, a 95% efficient inverter, what would be the expected ac output if 1000W/m² irradiance?

   a. 84.8kW to 87.4kW

   b. 100kW to 200kW

   c. 87.4kW to 90kW

   d. 88.7kW to 81.4kW

28. A 12V light is left on for 13 hours at 1.5A with a 12V battery. How much energy is used?

   a. 23 Ah

   b. 0.234 kWh

   c. 23.4 Wh

   d. 19.5 Ah

29. In the question above, how many Ah are used?

   a. 23 Ah

   b. 0.234 kWh

   c. 23.4 Wh

   d. 19.5 Ah

30. Electrical safety is best studied at

   a. OSHA website

   b. OSH website

   c. CSLB website

   d. UL website

31. The interconnection of a PV system is approved by

   a. City

   b. County

   c. State

   d. Utility

32. Grounding (bonding) of a transformerless PV system on a roof should be done to
   a. Stainless-steel hardware
   b. Flashings
   c. Racking and aluminum frames
   d. Grounded conductor

33. Lowest grid voltage
   a. Transmission
   b. Distribution
   c. Service equipment
   d. Generation

34. If a 12V PV module has 36 cells, then how many volts is a 54-cell module?
   a. 6V
   b. 18V
   c. 24V
   d. 17V

35. Transformers convert
   a. High voltage low current to low voltage low current
   b. Low voltage low current to high voltage high current
   c. High voltage low current to low voltage high current
   d. Low current low current to high voltage low current

36. Undersized PV array
   a. Decreases voltage drop
   b. Decreases battery life
   c. Increases current drop
   d. Increases resistance

37. Bypass diodes
   a. Reduce current
   b. Limit effects of shading
   c. Are wired in series with groups of solar cells and prevent reverse current
   d. Are in the combiner box

38. Microinverters are connected between the _____ and the _____.

    a. PV module, service panel

    b. String, combiner

    c. Main breaker, backfeed breaker

    d. Utility meter, transformer

39. A system that sits on a flat/low slope rooftop and has no penetrations is called a

    a. Flush mounted system

    b. Flashed system

    c. BIPV system

    d. Ballasted system

40. What is the proper slope of an extension ladder?

    a. 1:3

    b. 1:4

    c. 1:5

    d. 1:6

41. Voc = 22V, Vmp = 18V, hot PV cell temp = 50°C, inverter operating voltage range = 250V to 600V, temp coefficient of voltage = − 0.38%/°C. What is the LEAST amount of PV modules that should be connected in series?

    a. 12

    b. 14

    c. 16

    d. 18

42. The primary power source for a utility interactive PV system is the

    a. Inverter

    b. Utility

    c. PV

    d. Charge controller

Figure 12.1 IV curve

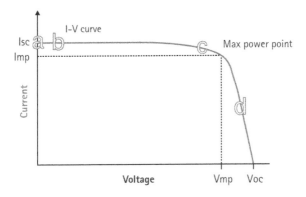

43. Which place on the IV curve in Figure 12.1 produces power and has the most current?

    a. A

    b. B

    c. C

    d. D

44. What is specified on a charge controller

    a. Irradiance limit

    b. Insolation limit

    c. Maximum voltage

    d. Minimum current

45. Units for irradiance are
   a. Energy per area
   b. Power per area
   c. Volts per square meter
   d. Amps per square meter

46. What is used to calculate maximum system voltage?
   a. Current
   b. Power
   c. Temperature
   d. Irradiance

47. What will be increased by reflective surfaces (albedo)?
   a. Voltage
   b. Resistance
   c. Current
   d. AM

For the following 3 questions, use the information from Table 12.1.

Table 12.1 Table for questions 48 to 50

Power	250W
Open Circuit Voltage	40V
Maximum Power Voltage	35V
Short Circuit Current	8A
Maximum Power Current	7.14A
Temp Coefficient for Voltage	−0.33%/°C
CEC Power	220W
NOCT	48°C
Inverter low MPPT voltage	230V
Inverter maximum input voltage	550V

48. There are 4 PV source circuits of 10 modules each. What is the MPPT voltage of the array at Standard Test Conditions?

    a. 160V

    b. 350V

    c. 140V

    d. 230V

49. What is the power of the array?

    a. 10kW

    b. 110kW

    c. 1000W

    d. 40kW

50. What is the maximum number of modules in series at a location with a low temperature of minus 40°C?

    a. 9

    b. 10

    c. 11

    d. 12

51. What is the best voltage for charging a 12V lead-acid battery?

    a. 12V

    b. 11.8V

    c. 12.3V

    d. 14.1V

52. Unit for resistance?

    a. Amp

    b. Volt

    c. Om

    d. Ohm

53. Wind uplift forces in the construction industry in the US are measured in

    a. Pounds per square foot

    b. Miles per hour

    c. Square feet per pound

    d. kW per m^2

54. Direction on a compass is
   a. Latitude
   b. Longitude
   c. Meridian
   d. Azimuth

55. Hydraulic analogy for voltage is
   a. Pressure
   b. Flow
   c. Volume
   d. Drag

56. Which room cannot have a PV dc disconnect?
   a. Kitchen
   b. Attic
   c. Bathroom
   d. Bedroom

57. Stand-alone inverter output goes to
   a. Loads
   b. Utility
   c. Meter
   d. PV

58. Best sealant for residential rooftop
   a. Polyurethane
   b. Paraffin
   c. Bitumen
   d. Silicon

59. 500W/m^2 for 4 hours is
   a. 20kWh/m^2
   b. 2kWh/m^2
   c. 2kW/m^2
   d. 5kW

60. For a supply side connection, the output of the inverter is limited by
   a. Service entrance conductor ampacity
   b. Load side breaker ampacity
   c. PV dimension and quantity
   d. Locational irradiance

61. Which is the smallest installable part of a PV system?
   a. Solar panel
   b. Solar module
   c. Solar array
   d. PV source circuit

62. What is the most typical hazard with PV systems of the following?
   a. Shock
   b. Arc flash
   c. Lightning
   d. Earthquake

63. A 4kW PV system with 15% losses in a location with 4.5 sun hours per day, what would be the annual output?
   a. 985.5kWh
   b. 1450kWh
   c. 5585kWh
   d. 4550kWh

64. If available roof area is 12m^2 and the PV is 15% efficient, then how much PV will fit?
   a. 4.5kW
   b. 2.2kW
   c. 1.8kW
   d. 3.3kW

65. Which of the following is a typical direct PV system application?
   a. Lighting
   b. Batteries
   c. Pumping water
   d. Fire alarm

66. Current is affected mostly by
   a. The number of solar cells in series
   b. The size of the solar cell
   c. The backsheet of the solar module
   d. The temperature of the cell

67. In California (east of the zero-degree isogonic line) the north needle of the compass will point
   a. East of true North
   b. West of true North
   c. North of true North
   d. South of true North

68. Maintenance of sealed valve regulated lead acid batteries includes
   a. Checking fluid levels
   b. Equalization charge
   c. Scrubbing lead plates
   d. Cleaning terminals

69. Given that Voc is 18V and the temperature correction factor = 1.2. What would be the maximum system voltage if there were 16 modules in series?
   a. 340V
   b. 346V
   c. 240V
   d. 440V

70. STC watts can be calculated by
   a. Vmp × Voc
   b. Voc × Isc
   c. Vmp × Imp
   d. PTC × CEC

ANSWERS

1. An off-grid installation has a 1HP pump that is on 10% of the time and a 20W light that is on 100% of the time. What is the energy use per month?
   a. 54Wh
   b. 68kW
   c. 68kWh
   d. 0.63 MWh

Question 1 is **c**
1HP = 746W
746W × 0.1 × 24hrs × 30 days = 53,712Wh
20W × 24hr × 30 days = 14,400Wh
53,712Wh + 14,400Wh = 68,112Wh
68,112Wh/1000 = **68kWh**
Discussion: NABCEP requires you know that 746W = 1 horsepower (HP). Often pumps are rated in horsepower. These are typical load energy calculations and you should be comfortable converting units and performing energy calculations when given power and time.

2. What kind of ground faults do most inverters detect?
   a. High voltage
   b. Medium voltage
   c. Ac
   d. Dc

Question 2 is **d**
Inverters detect dc ground faults
Discussion: Ac ground faults are detected on the ac side of the inverter often at a distribution panel, i.e., main service panel, load center or switchgear. Most inverters are not connected to high or medium voltage. Medium voltage is thousands of volts, by most definitions and large utility scale inverters are often connected to medium voltage via a transformer.

3. Current carrying ability of a conductor (wire) is called
   a. Ampacity
   b. Amps
   c. Inductance
   d. Insolation

Question 3 is **a**
Current carrying ability is ampacity.

4. According to Ohm's Law and voltage drop, the relationship between voltage drop and current is
   a. Proportional
   b. Inversely proportional
   c. Directly inverse
   d. Inversely direct

Question 4 is **a**
Ohm's Law states: $V = IR$
If I goes up and R remains constant, then V goes up. You can also remember that with voltage drop, more current makes more voltage drop. **Voltage and current are proportional**. This is one reason why we need a larger wire with more current, so the wire resistance is less with a larger wire and there will be less voltage drop.

5. An Array in Sacramento California in August (hot and dry) is not producing as expected. Which of the following is NOT a likely problem?
   a. Decreased ac wire size and voltage loss
   b. String size too short
   c. String size too long
   d. Soiling

Question 5 is **c**
Late summer in Sacramento is hot and can be dry. When it is hot, voltage can be low. **Too long of a string would be a problem when it is too cold**, not hot. Soiling could be a problem, since in a dry place, there can be dust without rain to wash it away. Pay attention to the word NOT in a question. Also, since there are two answers that are opposites, there is a good chance that one of them is the correct answer.

6. When using a digital multimeter, what is the first thing you should do?

    a. Turn the meter on

    b. Inspect the meter

    c. Touch the black lead to the white wire

    d. Touch the black lead to the black wire

Question 6 is **b**

Always inspect first. When taking an exam always think on the safe side. Look before you touch. Often safety questions are easy.

7. Which is the worst design error?

    a. BIPV on a commercial job

    b. A fast growing tree to the north of the array in Idaho

    c. PV at 5-degree tilt at 40 degrees latitude

    d. Different tilt angles in a PV source circuit

Question 7 is **d**

Different tilt or azimuth orientation within a source circuit is bad. **Series connections should not have different orientations**.

8. The low design temperature is $-20°C$ and the Voc temperature correction factor for your PV is $-0.34\%/°C$. The characteristics of your module are Isc = 8A, Voc = 37V and Vmp = 29V. How many modules can you put in series for an inverter that cannot go over 500V?

    a. 10

    b. 11

    c. 12

    d. 13

Question 8 is **b**

$-20°C - 25°C = -45°C$

$-45°C \times -0.34\%/°C = 15.3\%$ increase Voc

$1.15 \times 37Voc = 42.6V$ cold

$500V/42.6V = 11.7$

Round down to **11 in series**

Rounding up would bring the voltage over the inverter limit.

9. MPPT is for
  a. Optimizing energy from the utility
  b. Getting the most energy from a battery with a MPPT inverter
  c. Optimizing power from a PV array
  d. Tracking the sun with a 2-axis tracker

Question 9 is **c**
MPPT is maximum power point tracking and will **optimize the energy harnessed from PV**. Some inverters have multiple MPPTs. Charge controllers often, but not always have MPPTs.

10. Concentrated PV
  a. Only works with direct sunlight
  b. Usually has a single axis tracker
  c. Will get 30% power during cloudy conditions
  d. Is using heat to make electricity

Question 10 is **a**
Concentrated PV only works with direct sunlight. Also concentrated PV usually works with 2-axis trackers that always point at the sun and will not work at all during cloudy conditions. We need direct sunlight, so we can focus sunbeams to make concentrating solar technologies work. Many people confuse concentrating PV with concentrating solar thermal. PV is converting sunlight directly to electricity, whereas thermal is working with heat.

11. Fall protection should be used at heights over
  a. 4 feet
  b. 2 feet
  c. 3 feet
  d. 6 feet

Question 11 is **d**
Fall protection required over 6 feet. If you are in another country, you probably are required to have fall protection at heights over 2 meters, which is slightly more than 6 feet.

12. Parallel PV circuit connections increase
   a. Voltage
   b. Current
   c. Resistance
   d. EMF

Question 12 is **b**
Parallel connections increase current. Series increases voltage.

13. Optimal tilt for off-grid PV system in the winter
   a. Latitude
   b. Latitude −15 degrees
   c. Latitude +15 degrees
   d. Vertical

Question 13 is **c**
Optimal tilt to maximize winter production is latitude +15 degrees. The sun is lower in the winter, which requires a higher tilt angle.

14. What is the most acceptable rating of an enclosure for exposed circuit conductors mounted on an outside wall?
   a. NEMA 3R
   b. NEMA 11
   c. NEMA 4X
   d. NEMA 12

Question 14 is **a**
Typically, NEMA 3 and NEMA 3R enclosures are used outside. Often there will be a NEMA 3 disconnect on the outside of a building. Take a look the next time you pass a disconnect. NEMA stands for National Equipment Manufacturers Association.

15. Bypass diodes are located in the
   a. Combiner box
   b. Inverter
   c. Wiring harness
   d. PV module

Question 15 is **d**

Bypass diodes are in PV module junction box. Bypass diodes till divert current around a group of solar cells if there is a shaded solar cell in that group. There are often 3 bypass diodes per PV module.

16. A PV array at a higher elevation would tend to produce more
   a. Current
   b. Heat
   c. Resistance
   d. Polysilicon

Question 16 is **a**

Higher elevation = less atmosphere = more irradiance = **more current**. Higher elevations can also be cooler and you can have more voltage from cold temperatures.

17. Voc = 36V, low temp = − 2°C, inverter maximum input voltage = 500V, temp coefficient of voltage = − 0.35%/°C. What is the maximum number of modules that can be connected in series?
   a. 13
   b. 10
   c. 11
   d. 12

Question 17 is **d**

− 2°C − 25°C = − 27°C

− 27°C × − 0.35%/°C = 9.45% increase Voc

1.0945 × 36Voc = 39.4Voc cold

500V/39.4V = 12.7

round down to **12 in series**

You can do these calculations different ways and come up with the same correct answer.

18. How much 14% efficient PV fits on 25 square meters?

   a. 3000W

   b. 4.5kW

   c. 4000W

   d. 3.5kW

Question 18 is **d**

14% efficient = $0.14 \times 1000W/m^2 = 140\ W/m^2$

$140W/m^2 \times 25\ m^2 = 3500W = \mathbf{3.5kW}$

19. Which is the smallest conductor?

   a. 18 AWG

   b. 10 AWG

   c. 0 AWG

   d. 3/0 AWG

Question 19 is **a**

18 AWG is the smallest conductor. From small to large the conductors listed are 18AWG, 10AWG, 0 AWG, 3/0 AWG. 0 AWG is also called 1/0 AWG. Most of the world does not use AWG (American Wire Gauge) wire sizes and uses a very simple to understand system. Most of the world uses the cross-sectional area of a conductor in square millimetres. For example, a 10AWG wire is 5.26 mm^2

20. Which of the following is the simplest type of PV system?

   a. Utility interactive

   b. Stand-alone

   c. Self-regulating

   d. Direct coupled

Question 20 is **d**

Direct coupled is the simplest and is just PV and a load that only works when the sun is out. Some would argue that a water pumping system could get complicated, since water systems can be complicated, but the PV part of these kinds of systems are the least complex.

21. Sun path charts differ based on
   a. Longitude
   b. Latitude
   c. Azimuth
   d. Tilt angle

Question 21 is **b**
Sun charts are specific for different latitudes (latitude = degrees from equator). Every place in the world that has the same latitude around the world will have the exact same sun path.

22. Series connections increase
   a. Voltage
   b. Current
   c. Cold
   d. Heat

Question 22 is **a**
Series increases voltage. Parallel increases current.

23. The longest shadow at 2PM would be on
   a. June 1
   b. November 12
   c. February 14
   d. March 29

Question 23 is **b**
The day closest to winter solstice (about 12/21) will have the longest shadow. The time of day is a distraction.

24. What is the ground mount advantage over a rooftop system?
   a. Takes no extra real estate
   b. Cooler
   c. Increased photosynthesis
   d. Soiling

Question 24 is **b**
A ground mount is **cooler** than a rooftop because of better airflow and will have higher voltage. Ground mounts take up more real estate and can get dirty (soiling) more easily near the dirt. Photosynthesis is how plants get energy from sunlight.

25. Which test conditions have higher voltage?
   a. STC
   b. PTC
   c. CEC
   d. NOCT

Question 25 is **a**
STC is higher voltage. The other test conditions listed have higher cell temperatures and lower voltage. The ambient temperature is always cooler than the cell temperature, because sunlight heats up solar cells often 30 degrees C over ambient on a sunny day.

26. Which is the best tilt angle for annual production in most of the USA (temperate latitudes)?
   a. Latitude +15 degrees
   b. Latitude −15 degrees
   c. 30 degrees
   d. Longitude tilt

Question 26 is **c**
Best tilt for most of the USA for annual production is about **30 degrees**. Most of the US is between latitudes of 30 and 40. Often a little less than latitude tilt is best for most of these places. Many of the populated areas around the world, including much of Europe, China and Japan, are in these latitudes and would have similar requirements for tilt. Tilt angles do not always have to be exact to be a good investment.

27. A 100kW STC PV system with 8% system losses, using PV that is +3 – 0% production tolerance, a 95% efficient inverter, what would be the expected ac output if 1000W/m² irradiance?

   a. 84.8kW to 87.4kW

   b. 100kW to 200kW

   c. 87.4kW to 90kW

   d. 88.7kW to 81.4kW

Question 27 is **c**

100kW × 0.92 × 1 × 0.95 = **87.4kW**

100kW × 0.92 × 1.03 × 0.95 = **90kW**

For +3 – 0% production tolerance the derating factor is 1 to 1.03. Many designers only look at the low end of the tolerance and would just give you the answer of 87.4kW, but if an answer has a range, go with both sides of the range for the correct answer.

28. A 12V light is left on for 13 hours at 1.5A with a 12V battery. How much energy is used?

   a. 23 Ah

   b. 0.234 kWh

   c. 23.4 Wh

   d. 19.5 Ah

Question 28 is **b**

12V × 1.5A × 13hr = 234Wh

234Wh/1000 = **0.234kWh**

29. In the question above, how many Ah are used?

   a. 23 Ah

   b. 0.234 kWh

   c. 23.4 Wh

   d. 19.5 Ah

Question 29 is **d**

1.5A × 13hrs = **19.5 Ah**

30. Electrical safety is best studied at
   a. OSHA website
   b. OSH website
   c. CSLB website
   d. UL website

Question 30 is **a**
Occupational Safety and Health Administration (**OSHA**) is for workplace safety including electrical safety.

31. The interconnection of a PV system is approved by
   a. City
   b. County
   c. State
   d. Utility

Question 31 is **d**
Interconnection is approved by the utility.

32. Grounding (bonding) of a transformerless PV system on a roof should be done to
   a. Stainless-steel hardware
   b. Flashings
   c. Racking and aluminum frames
   d. Grounded conductor

Question 32 is **c**
Racking and frames should be grounded (bonded) on every PV system. Stainless-steel hardware refers to nuts and bolts.

33. Lowest grid voltage
   a. Transmission
   b. Distribution
   c. Service equipment
   d. Generation

Question 33 is **c**
Service has the lowest voltage. Service voltage is the voltage at the building where the electricity is served.

34. If a 12V PV module has 36 cells, then how many volts is a 54-cell module?

    a. 6V

    b. 18V

    c. 24V

    d. 17V

Question 34 is **b**

12V/36 cells = 0.333V/cell

0.333V/cell × 54 cells = **18V**

35. Transformers convert

    a. High voltage low current to low voltage low current

    b. Low voltage low current to high voltage high current

    c. High voltage low current to low voltage high current

    d. Low current low current to high voltage low current

Question 35 is **c**

Transformers convert **high voltage low current to low voltage high current** (or vice versa). Since voltage times current is power, then we will have voltage go up and current go down or vice versa when comparing one side to the other.

36. Undersized PV array

    a. Decreases voltage drop

    b. Decreases battery life

    c. Increases current drop

    d. Increases resistance

Question 36 is **b**

Decreased array size decreases battery life (due to not charging battery fully). Not fully charging a battery is not good for the battery.

37. Bypass diodes
   a. Reduce current
   b. Limit effects of shading
   c. Are wired in series with groups of solar cells and prevent reverse current
   d. Are in the combiner box

Question 37 is **b**

Bypass diodes reduce effects of shading and are wired in parallel in cells in the junction box on the back of the PV module.

38. Microinverters are connected between the _____ and the _____.
   a. PV module, service panel
   b. String, combiner
   c. Main breaker, backfeed breaker
   d. Utility meter, transformer

Question 38 is **a**

Microinverters (and other **inverters**) are **between the PV and the service panel**.

39. A system that sits on a flat/low slope rooftop and has no penetrations is called a
   a. Flush mounted system
   b. Flashed system
   c. BIPV system
   d. Ballasted system

Question 39 is **d**

Ballasted systems are common fat low slope (fat) roof systems that are not penetrating the roof. A ballast is something that is relatively heavy keeps the PV from blowing away.

40. What is the proper slope of an extension ladder?

    a. 1:3

    b. 1:4

    c. 1:5

    d. 1:6

Question 40 is **b**

1:4 slope is required for a ladder according to OSHA. This means that for every 1 unit of distance towards you, the ladder will go up 4 units of distance. Many people who use ladders say that if you are standing with your feet at the base of a ladder and put your arms straight in front of you, if they touch the ladder, that is about a 1:4 slope.

41. V_{oc} = 22V, V_{mp} = 18V, hot PV cell temp = 50°C, inverter operating voltage range = 250V to 600V, temp coefficient of voltage = − 0.38%/°C. What is the LEAST amount of modules that should be connected in series?

    a. 12

    b. 14

    c. 16

    d. 18

Question 41 is **c**

Take note here that we are calculating the least number of modules in series and we are not performing a cold temperature maximum number in series calculation with V_{oc}. We will be determining the least number in series to perform correctly at V_{mp} on a hot day. The information we will need is the high cell temperature, the temperature coefficient of V_{mp}, V_{mp} and the lowest voltage for proper efficient operation. In this case we will calculate how much our voltage goes down, not how much it will go up. If you are taking the NABCEP Associate exam, you could expect this to be the most missed question on the exam.

50°C − 25°C = 25°C

25°C × − 0.38%/°C = 9.5% decrease in voltage

1 − 0.095 = 0.905

0.905 × 18V_{mp} = 16.3V_{mp} hot

250V/16.3V_{mp} = 15.3

Round up to **16 in series**

If you round down for hot temperatures you would not have enough voltage, so round up for hot and round down for cold. Having more voltage keeps you inside the voltage window on a hot day.

For hot voltage calculations, do not use V_{oc}, use V_{mp}. Use V_{oc} for cold calculations.

42. The primary power source for a utility interactive PV system is the

    a. Inverter

    b. Utility

    c. PV

    d. Charge controller

Question 42 is **b**

The **primary power source** for a **utility interactive** system is the **utility**. The interactive inverter will match the voltage and frequency of the utility.

Interesting note: Some off-grid systems will operate with multiple inverters and one of the inverters will be the master inverter, which determines the frequency and the other inverter(s) will follow the master inverter.

Figure 12.2 IV curve – answer

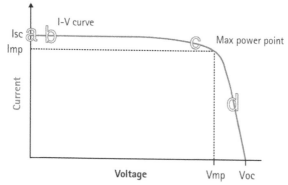

43. Which place on the IV curve in Figure 12.1 produces power and has the most current?

    a. A

    b. B

    c. C

    d. D

Question 43 is **b**

A is the most current, but produces no power and **b is the next most amount of current and produces power** (c produces the most power and d is the most voltage). See Figure 12.2.

44. What is specified on a charge controller
   a. Irradiance limit
   b. Insolation limit
   c. Maximum voltage
   d. Minimum current

Question 44 is **c**
A charge controller will have **maximum voltage specified** (and so will most any equipment). A charge controller will also specify maximum current.

45. Units for irradiance are
   a. Energy per area
   b. Power per area
   c. Volts per square meter
   d. Amps per square meter

Question 45 is **b**
Irradiance is power per area, usually measured in watts per square meter. 1000W/m² is the irradiance level called "peak sun" or irradiance at Standard Test Conditions. Energy per area is irradiation or insolation.

46. What is used to calculate maximum system voltage?
   a. Current
   b. Power
   c. Temperature
   d. Irradiance

Question 46 is **c**
Temperature is used to calculate maximum system voltage along with Voc, the temperature coefficient of Voc and the number of PV modules connected in series.

47 What will be increased by reflective surfaces (albedo)?
  a. Voltage
  b. Resistance
  c. Current
  d. AM

Question 47 is **c**

Reflections and increased light increases current. Reflected light can also be called **albedo**.

For the following 3 questions, use the information from Table 12.1.

Table 12.1 Table for questions 48 to 50

Power	250W
Open Circuit Voltage	40V
Maximum Power Voltage	35V
Short Circuit Current	8A
Maximum Power Current	7.14A
Temp Coefficient for Voltage	−0.33%/°C
CEC Power	220W
NOCT	48°C
Inverter low MPPT voltage	230V
Inverter maximum input voltage	550V

48. There are 4 PV source circuits of 10 modules each. What is the MPPT voltage of the array at Standard Test Conditions?
  a. 160V
  b. 350V
  c. 140V
  d. 230V

Question 48 is **b**

35Vmp × 10 in series = 350Vmp

Discussion. At STC an inverter should operate at Vmp for each module. If there are 10 PV modules in series, then 10 times Vmp should be the voltage where the array will operate.

49. What is the power of the array?

   a. 10kW

   b. 110kW

   c. 1000W

   d. 40kW

Question 49 is **a**

250W module × 40 modules = 10,000W

10,000W = **10kW**

An easy trick is to convert the power of the PV module to kW immediately, so a 250W module would be 0.25kW; usually we just put the decimal in front. 4 PV source circuits of 10 each is 40 modules.

50. What is the maximum number of modules in series at a location with a low temperature of minus 40°C?

   a. 9

   b. 10

   c. 11

   d. 12

Question 50 is **c**

$- 40°C - 25°C = - 65°C$

$- 65°C × - 0.33\%/°C = 21.45\%$ increase in Voc

$1.2145 × 40V = 48.6V$

$550V/48.4V = 11.4$

11 in series max

51. What is the best voltage for charging a 12V lead-acid battery?

   a. 12V

   b. 11.8V

   c. 12.3V

   d. 14.1V

Question 51 is **d**

Best voltage for **charging a 12V battery is 14.1V** (best of the choices given). A 12V lead-acid battery will sit charged at 12.6V and often charge somewhere between 14 and 15V. If a 12V lead-acid battery is at 50% depth of discharge, it will measure about 12V.

52. Unit for resistance?

   a. Amp

   b. Volt

   c. Om

   d. Ohm

Question 52 is **d**

Resistance is measured in Ohms (Ω).

53. Wind uplift forces in the construction industry in the US are measured in

   a. Pounds per square foot

   b. Miles per hour

   c. Square feet per pound

   d. kW per m^2

Question 53 is **a**

Wind uplift is measured in pounds per square foot (psf) in the US.

54. Direction on a compass is

   a. Latitude

   b. Longitude

   c. Meridian

   d. Azimuth

Question 54 is **d**

Direction on a compass is azimuth. Latitude is degrees from the equator.

55. Hydraulic analogy for voltage is

   a. Pressure

   b. Flow

   c. Volume

   d. Drag

Question 55 is **a**

Hydraulic analogy for voltage is pressure. Current is flow.

56. Which room cannot have a PV dc disconnect?

    a. Kitchen

    b. Attic

    c. Bathroom

    d. Bedroom

Question 56 is **c**

PV dc disconnect not allowed in bathroom (think of wet feet).

57. Stand-alone inverter output goes to

    a. Loads

    b. Utility

    c. Meter

    d. PV

Question 57 is **a**

Off-grid inverter output goes to loads. Loads are what use electricity.

58. Best sealant for residential rooftop

    a. Polyurethane

    b. Paraffin

    c. Bitumen

    d. Silicon

Question 58 is **a**

Polyurethane and silicone are the best sealants of the examples given. Silicone is a sealant silicon is what solar cells are made of. There is a big difference.

59. $500W/m^2$ for 4 hours is

    a. $20kWh/m^2$

    b. $2kWh/m^2$

    c. $2kW/m^2$

    d. $5kW$

Question 59 is **b**

$500W/m^2 \times 4$ hours = **2kWh**

60. For a supply side connection, the output of the inverter is limited by
  a. Service entrance conductor ampacity
  b. Load side breaker ampacity
  c. PV dimension and quantity
  d. Locational irradiance

Question 60 is **a**

Supply side inverter output is **limited by the service entrance conductors**. The loads are already protected from the utility by the main service disconnect (main breaker).

61. Which is the smallest installable part of a PV system?
  a. Solar panel
  b. Solar module
  c. Solar array
  d. PV source circuit

Question 61 is **b**.

A solar module is the smallest unit that you can install. A solar panel is made up of solar modules. You cannot install a single solar cell, a number of solar cells are put together to make a module. Most modules have 60 or 72 cells.

62. What is the most typical hazard with PV systems of the following?
  a. Shock
  b. Arc flash
  c. Lightning
  d. Earthquake

Question 62 is **a**.

Solar installers are always concerned about shocks and falls. Arc flashes can be very dangerous, but are less common than shocks.

63. A 4kW PV system with 15% losses in a location with 4.5 sun hours per day, what would be the annual output?

- **a.** 985.5kWh
- **b.** 1450kWh
- **c.** 5585kWh
- **d.** 4550kWh

Question 63 is **c**.

4kW × 0.85 × 4.5 sun hours × 365 days = 5585kWh

Discussion: Losing 15% means keeping 85%, which is where the 0.85 derating factor comes from. Always think about what you keep. With this kind of question, look at the information that you are given and then make logical use of the information. Do not get distracted if you see a derating factor that you are not used to.

64. If available roof area is 12m² and the PV is 15% efficient, then how much PV will fit?

- **a.** 4.5kW
- **b.** 2.2kW
- **c.** 1.8kW
- **d.** 3.3kW

Question 64 is **c**.

15% efficient PV is 15% of 1000W/m²

$0.15 \times 1000W/m^2 = 150W/m^2$

$150W/m^2 \times 12m^2 = 1800W$

$1800W/1000 = \textbf{1.8kW}$

65. Which of the following is a typical direct PV system application?

- **a.** Lighting
- **b.** Batteries
- **c.** Pumping water
- **d.** Fire alarm

Question 65 is **c**.

Pumping water is a common direct-coupled PV application. A water pump motor hooked up to PV with no inverter or battery is a direct system. When the sun shines, the pump will pump. Water can be stored at a height, so that water pressure can be had at night.

66. Current is affected mostly by
   a. The number of solar cells in series
   b. The size of the solar cell
   c. The backsheet of the solar module
   d. The temperature of the cell

Question 66 is **b**.

The size of the solar cell determines the current of a PV module. A larger solar cell will capture more photons and convert them to electron flow. The number of cells in series determines the voltage.

67. In California (east of the zero-degree isogonic line) the north needle of the compass will point
   a. East of true North
   b. West of true North
   c. North of true North
   d. South of true North

In California, magnetic declination is to the east. This means that the north end of the compass will point slightly to the east.

68. Maintenance of sealed valve regulated lead-acid batteries includes
   a. Checking fluid levels
   b. Equalization charge
   c. Scrubbing lead plates
   d. Cleaning terminals

Question 68 is **d**.

On a **sealed** lead-acid battery (also known as maintenance free), one does not have access to the electrolyte fluids. Equalization is not done on sealed batteries, since equilization requires distilled water to be added to the battery. All batteries can have their terminals cleaned.

69. Given that Voc is 18V and the temperature correction factor for voltage = 1.2. What would be the maximum system voltage if there were 16 modules in series?

   a. 340V

   b. 346V

   c. 240V

   d. 440V

Questivon 69 is **b**.

18V × 1.2 correction factor × 16 in series = 346V

70. STC watts can be calculated by

   a. Vmp × Voc

   b. Voc × Isc

   c. Vmp × Imp

   d. PTC × CEC

Question 70 is **c**.

Vmp × Imp = STC watts

At Voc there is no current and power is zero. At Isc there is no voltage and power is zero.

When taking an exam, the best way to perform well is by being prepared, calm, confident and well rested. Good luck!

Sean White

CHAPTER 3 PV MATH ANSWERS

1. A 200-watt light is left on for 7 days. How much energy is consumed?
  a. 34kWh
  b. 336kW
  c. 3360Wh
  d. 14MWh

power × time = energy
200W × 24 hrs/day × 7 days = 33,600Wh
33,600Wh/1000W/kW = 33.6kWh
33.6kWh is closest to 34kWh
correct answer is a.

2. If a 100W light bulb is working on a 120V socket, what is the current?
  a. 12kW
  b. 0.83A
  c. 1.2A
  d. 144 Ω

volts × current = power (VI = P)
I = P/V
I = 100W/120V = 0.833A
correct answer is b.

3. How much resistance does the light bulb have in question 2 above?
  a. 0.83 ohms
  b. 12 ohms
  c. 0.007 Ω
  d. 144 Ω

volts = current × resistance (V = IR)
R = V/I
R = 120V/0.833A = 144Ω
correct answer is d.

4. The hydraulic analogy for voltage is
   a. Flow
   b. Volume
   c. Capacity
   d. Pressure

voltage is like pressure
correct answer is d.

5. The hydraulic analogy for current is
   a. Flow
   b. Volume
   c. Capacity
   d. Pressure

current is like flow
correct answer is a.

6. Current required to send one MW (million watts) at the voltage of one MV (million volts)?
   a. 1A
   b. 1 million Amperes
   c. 1Ah
   d. 100A

Volts x Amps = Watts
Amps = Watts/Volts
Amps = 1,000,000W/1,000,000V = 1A
This goes to show why high voltage is efficient for transporting electricity.
An Ampere is the same as an amp is abbreviated A.
correct answer is a.

7. 2000 watts is equal to
   a. 20kW
   b. 2kW
   c. 0.2kW
   d. 2kWh

kilo = 1000
1kW is 1000W, so 2kW is 2000W (move decimal 3 places).
Also, can divide by 1000 to move decimal 3 places.
correct answer is b.

8. The power of a 250-watt solar module is equal to
   a. 1/4th of a kW
   b. 0.025MW
   c. 25KVA
   d. 0.25kWh

move decimal 3 places to left to make watts kilowatts
250W/1000 = 0.25kW
250W = 0.250kW
0.25 =25%= ¼
correct answer is a.

9. One horsepower equals
   a. 0.746kW
   b. 746kWh
   c. 1000W
   d. 1MW

1 HP = 746W
746W/1000W/kW = 0.746kW (move decimal 3 places)
correct answer is a.

10. A pump works at 4A and 12V for 3 hours. How much energy does it consume?

   a. 144kWh

   b. 48Wh

   c. 0.144kWh

   d. 96Wh

Volts × Amps = Watts (V x A = W)

12V × 4A = 48W = Power

Power × Time = Energy

48W × 3 hours = 144Wh

144Wh/1000W/kW = 0.144kWh

correct answer is c.

Appendix 1

COMMON CONVERSIONS AND INTERPRETATIONS

National Electric Code = Code for wiring systems in the USA and other countries.

British Wiring Standard = Common "code" for the UK and many Commonwealth countries

Canadian Electric Code = Code for Canada

International Electrotechnical Commission (IEC) = Standard many countries' codes are aligned with around the world.

Wire sizing system in the USA = American Wire Gauge

Wire sizing system in most of world = cross sectional area in mm^2

Common PV wire size = 10AWG wire = 5.26 mm^2

Neutral wire color USA = White (or gray)

Neutral wire color International Electrotechnical Commission = Blue

2.54cm = 1 inch

1m = 3.28 feet

Residual Current Device (RCD) = Ground Fault Circuit Interrupter (GFCI)

Earthing = Grounding

Index

A reference in *italics* refers to a figure and references in **bold** show a table.